GARDEN YOUR WAY TO HEALTH AND FITNESS

GARDEN YOUR WAY TO HEALTH AND FITNESS

EXERCISE PLANS | INJURY PREVENTION | ERGONOMIC DESIGNS

BUNNY GUINNESS AND **JACQUELINE KNOX**

Timber Press
Portland • London

To Kevin, who expects little and gets less. B.G.
To my back-up team. J.K.

All photographs and illustrations by Bunny Guinness except those appearing on pages 17, 38, 41, 52, 70, 72, 74, 79–82, 87, 130–132, 159, 191 (upper), and 197 by Kevin M. R. Guinness; page 73 by Unity Guinness; pages 10, 14, 18–25, 26 (upper), 27, 31–33, 42, 47–51, 54–57, 59–61, 63, 66, 67 (upper), 75–77, 87 (right), 89–90, 109, 122–123, 124 (upper), 125, 142, 152, 158 (middle), 165, 177, 180–181, 186–188, 190, and 205–206 by Colin Leftley; pages 9, 12–13, 30, 46, 58, 65, 68–69, 98–100, 104, 111 (upper right), 118 (upper left and lower), 139 (lower), 145 (lower), 150 (upper), 157 (upper), 170–171, 193, 198, 201 (lower), and 202 by Marianne Majerus; and page 135 by Marie O'Hara.

Garden plan on pages 108–109 created by Bunny Guinness and coloured by Coral Mula.

Gardens designed by Bunny Guinness (pages 12–13, 29, 36–38, 44–46, 88, 92, 102–106, 109–110, 111 [upper left and lower left], 112–114, 115 [upper], 118 [upper left and lower], 119, 120 [middle and bottom], 121, 140–141, 150 [upper], 157, 158 [top], 160, 163–164, 170–171, 182–185, 189, and 204); Helen Dillon (pages 148 and 150 lower); Sarah Eberle (page 118 upper right); Val Jackson (page 94); Francesca Kendall (page 175); Ian and Susie Pasley-Taylor (page 107 upper), Mr. and Mrs. Shoji (pages 111 upper right and 178); Alexandre Thomas (120 top); and Cleve West (107 lower).

Mention of trademark, proprietary product, or vendor does not constitute a guarantee or warranty of the product by the publisher or authors and does not imply its approval to the exclusion of other products or vendors.

Before following any advice or practice suggested in this book, it is recommended that you consult your doctor as to its suitability, particularly if you suffer from any health problems or special conditions. The publishers, authors, and photographers cannot accept responsibility for any injuries or damage incurred as a result of following the exercises in this book, or of using any of the therapeutic techniques described or mentioned here.

Published in 2008 by Timber Press, Inc.

The Haseltine Building   2 The Quadrant
133 S.W. Second Avenue, Suite 450   135 Salusbury Road
Portland, Oregon 97204-3547, USA   London NW6 6RJ UK
www.timberpress.com   www.timberpress.co.uk

Designed by The Bridgewater Book Company
Printed in China

Library of Congress Cataloging-in-Publication Data
Guinness, Bunny.
Garden your way to health and fitness : / by Bunny Guinness & Jacqueline Knox.
p. cm.
Includes bibliographical references.
ISBN-13: 978-0-88192-881-5 (alk. paper)

1. Gardening. 2. Gardens–Design. 3. Gardening–Therapeutic use.
4. Health. 5. Exercises. I. Knox, Jacqueline. II. Title.

SB453.G895 2008 635--dc22 2007041869

A catalogue record for this book is also available from the British Library.

Contents

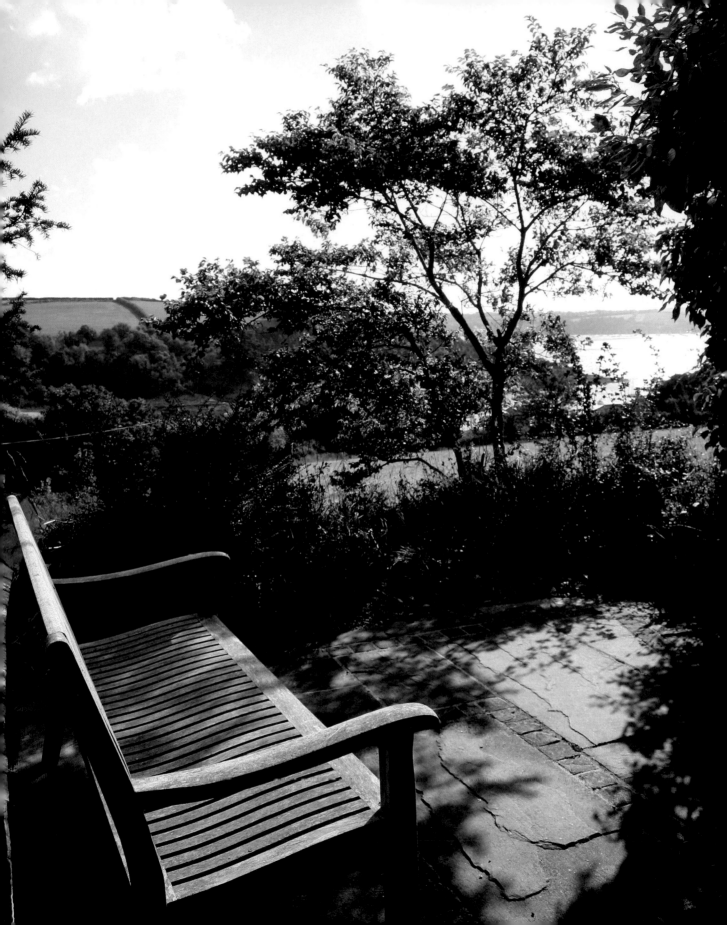

Introduction

Over the years, designing gardens for a diverse range of people has really brought home to me what extraordinary assets they can be. Gardens embellish our homes and landscapes, but perhaps even more important is the way they make us feel.

Conducive to soothing relaxation as well as dynamic activity, gardens stir our senses, enhance our emotional wellbeing, and improve our physical fitness. My own garden is no exception: it is where I go to gather my thoughts as I start the day and unravel a scrambled, stressed brain at the end of it. On red-letter occasions when I get to spend the whole day out there, I feel supercharged yet totally relaxed by nightfall.

A doctor once told me that gardeners live longer. I suspect he was sharing a personal observation rather than citing scientific research, but I do believe this notion must hold some grain of truth. In my experience, working in the garden can work wonders for one's health.

Gardening is certainly a foil to lethargy; rather than sitting in front of the television or surfing the internet, being involved with our gardens means there is always something egging us on—a plant that we want to take cuttings from to increase stock, a grapevine that needs pruning, or a hungry bird that is clamouring for food.

Once we get on our feet and venture outside we become carried away, immersed in other fruitful and absorbing tasks as our bodies and minds reap the benefits of being in the fresh air and lush surroundings. Stresses and worries peel away as the body loosens up through physical activity. Breathing becomes deeper, the scents lift our moods, and we lose ourselves in the movements—sometimes gentle and slow, sometimes thoroughly sweat-inducing—that make up our gardening routines.

Any person, of any age, can reap benefits. There has been much talk these days of children having 'nature deficit disorder', but if they get into the habit of playing outdoors and engaging with nature from a young age, it becomes habitual and they grow to enjoy running on the lawn, building forts in woodland clearings and playing imaginary games outside rather than lounging about in front of a video. At the other end of the spectrum, older gardeners who are less active than they once were can still benefit from tending plants in the fresh air, which is far better than being tucked up in a sedentary fashion indoors.

GARDENING SAFELY

While gardening has the potential to make us feel healthy and refreshed, it can also bring about soreness, stress, and strain. So many gardeners I know complain of aching backs and sore necks, and some even develop serious injuries from all the repetitive movement, twisting, and awkward bending that gardening can involve. While this is unfortunate, the good news is that this garden-related pain and injury is, to some degree, preventable; often, the solution lies in how we treat our bodies when we garden.

Since meeting Jacqueline Knox, physiotherapist and Pilates expert, I have grown to understand the importance of looking after my body in the garden. I had been studying Pilates as a way to keep fit, lean, and toned, and in time Jacky and I started to explore how the body-balancing techniques I learned in the Pilates studio could be applied out in the garden. Her approach is very simple: she recommends taking a few minutes to balance, centre, and strengthen our bodies before gardening; carrying out gardening tasks in a way that lessens the risk of injury while maximizing fitness benefits; and doing a series of stretches—tailormade to benefit gardeners—after gardening. By following Jacky's advice, and also through my own long process of learning what works best, I now feel loosened up and thoroughly energized, rather than spent and sore, after a few hours in the garden.

Gardening is, after all, a process of trial and error. If something does not quite work, we experiment with ways to change it. So, too, with the physical element of working in the garden: if reaching in a certain way causes us shoulder pain, it makes sense to take steps to change this action until we get it right. Throughout the second half of the book, step-by-step instructions for correctly carrying garden maintenance tasks like weeding, hoeing, and pushing a wheelbarrow are provided. Following these guidelines, combined with Jacky's advice on stretching, balancing the body, and warming up, should bring about a real improvement in how gardening makes you feel. Wearing the right clothing, choosing ergonomic tools, and understanding how to prevent and treat common gardeners' ailments (described in Chapter 3) can help us to tend to our bodies just as carefully as we tend to our landscapes.

Exercise in the garden can take many forms (some more dangerous than others)!

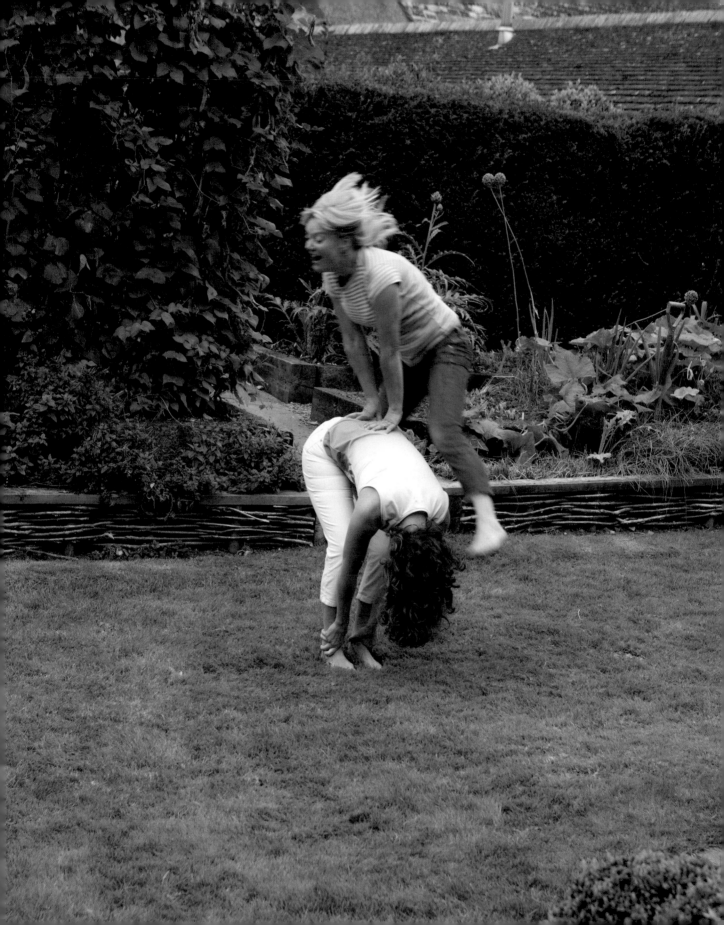

A VIABLE ALTERNATIVE TO THE GYM

Most of us experiment with a range of sports and exercise routines during the course of our lives.We might try a gym-based activity, cycling, a team sport, or jogging. Often, activities like these lose their appeal as our commitment levels gradually ease off or disappear.

Gardening is different. It engages our creative focus, and is intensely rewarding. Working in my garden never bores me: the varied activity keeps me on my toes and makes me think (what can I do here? why is this plant doing that?), yet it is also highly restful and therapeutic. I find that even the most cautious first-time gardeners become hooked after a very short time, because

they not only feel fantastic after a satisfying day spent in their plot but also have 'something to show for it'. That 'something' will continue to improve as long as we keep up the tending and creating—and so gardening is an activity in which there is little risk of losing interest.

Many people may not realize that gardening can also be a truly formidable calorie burner. If we spend a Sunday morning in the garden, with an hour mowing the lawn and then an hour and a half weeding, we complete a serious workout, burning calories and avoiding a trip to the gym. And in addition to burning calories, garden maintenance techniques often require resistance movements that can really tone muscles. When we are regularly active in the garden, exercise ceases to be something we do in isolated spurts several times per week; instead, it becomes a sustainable part of our daily lifestyles.

By bringing portable exercise equipment into our gardens, we can turn them into 'outdoor gyms' to suit our fitness preference and supplement our gardening workouts. As we will see in Chapter 2, the garden is a great place to do aerobic exercises, work out with a weighted ball and foam rollers, do a Swiss Ball routine, or even construct an exercise beam or stretching post. After a session of dynamic gardening and exercise, it is relaxing to use the garden as a place to wind down, practising deep breathing in the fresh air.

THE FEEL GOOD FACTOR

In addition to its physical benefits, most gardeners find that creating a bit of personal space—installing pathways, creating flower borders, and designing with the 'green architecture' of trees and hedging—brings about

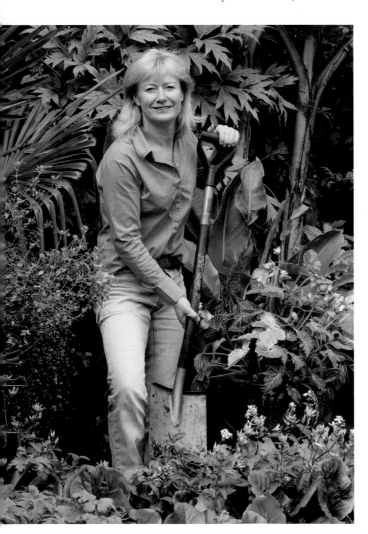

I love digging in the garden. It is satisfying work, and I really see results. The bonus is that it burns nearly 300 calories an hour.

real emotional rewards. I have seen gardeners who are depressed, recovering from illness, or less mobile than they once were, gaining huge benefit from designing and cultivating their own landscapes. Gardening seems to engender a sense of accomplishment which in turn boosts self-confidence and helps us to deal with other aspects of life.

This 'feel good factor' that active gardening brings about is well documented. Thirty minutes of aerobic exercise has been shown to improve mood in patients with major depression, and some studies have even suggested that exercise can delay or forestall some of the brain's aging processes and improve memory. With more strenuous activity the body releases adrenaline, along with endorphines like serotonin and dopamine, and these work together to enhance mood. The field of horticultural therapy, where patients suffering from physical or mental ailments use gardening as a tool for regaining a sense of control over their lives and beating depression, has been gaining popularity.

Simply being outside in the sunlight affects how we feel. In addition to the physiological benefits of light exposure (among other perks, it helps us to better absorb Vitamin D, which is good for bone strength), fresh air, and sunshine seem to have an intrinsically soothing effect. If you have young children, you will probably notice that if they suffer a minor injury like a bump on the knee indoors, being taken outside almost always makes them stop crying. It seems like magic, but it isn't: fresh air and greenery calm the senses, and when we are outdoors noises seem less intense and the stimulation of the natural landscape deflects attention from the minor things that vex us.

I highly recommend using your garden to unwind on a regular basis, whether this means strolling around with a cup of coffee each morning or just relaxing in a woodland clearing that overlooks a stunning view.

A GARDEN THAT WORKS FOR YOU

Even if you are hard-pressed for time you can still create a richly satisfying garden by choosing your plants and hard landscaping materials carefully. A high-maintenance garden has its positive points—among other pluses, the demands of trees, hedges and flower borders drive you to keep your mind and body active—but a more relaxed approach can still yield terrific, low-maintenance spaces.

The second half of the book explores a range of different strategies for creating a garden that demands only the amount of maintenance you are able to give to it and works in harmony with your health and fitness goals. Chapter 4 highlights various ways of using landscaping options like paving, gravel, steps, slopes, lawns, and pathways to create a garden that suits your activity level, whether you want to use the space for exercise, relaxation, or both. Planting schemes are a vital tool for personalizing your space, making it more attractive, private, and welcoming; in Chapter 5, I explain how to design borders geared towards various maintenance levels and explore ideas for using trees and hedging. Finally, in Chapter 6 I describe how to grow health-promoting fruits, vegetables, and herbs, highlighting those plants that will thrive with very little work.

The amazing thing about a garden is that it grows with you. The entire process is decidedly creative, and it is also thoroughly empowering: you can transform the look of a house, create wonderful useable spaces around it, cultivate foods, and restore your sanity by indulging in half an hour's absorbing physical work at the end of a fraught, office-bound day. If you can boost your health and avoid stresses and strains in the process, it becomes all the more satisfying. Whichever section you turn to first, and whether you decide to dip into this book once in a while or follow our advice religiously, just remember that gardening should never hurt; it should be fun, and the garden is *your* space. Enjoy!

Bunny Guinness

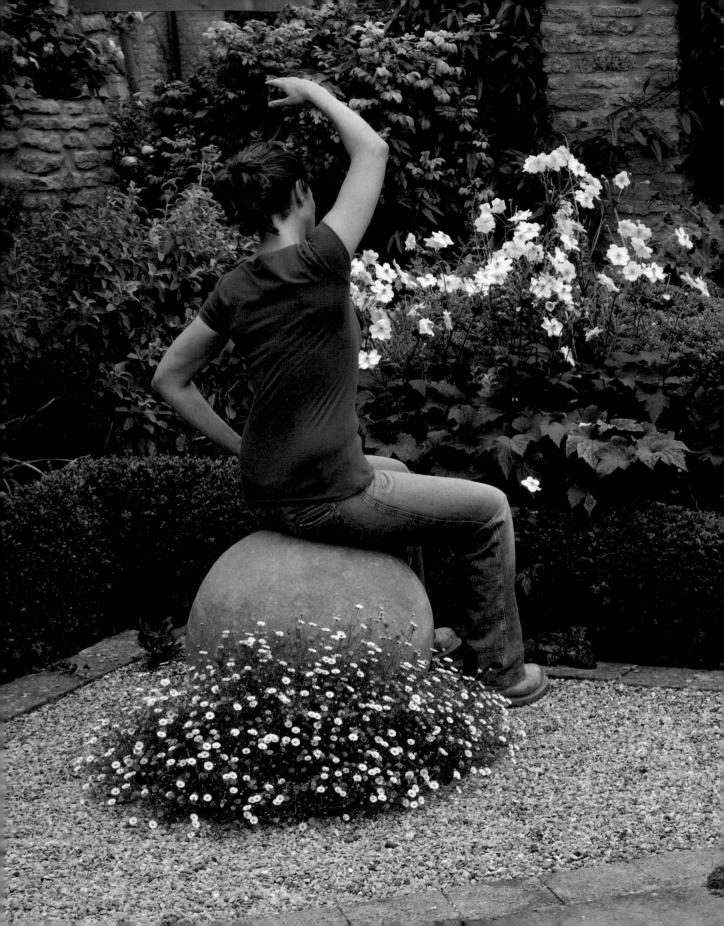

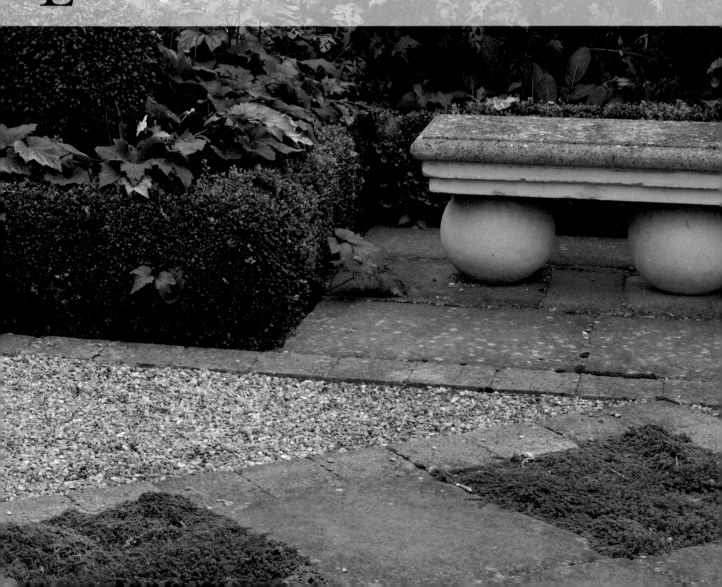

CHAPTER 1
ELEMENTS OF GARDEN FITNESS

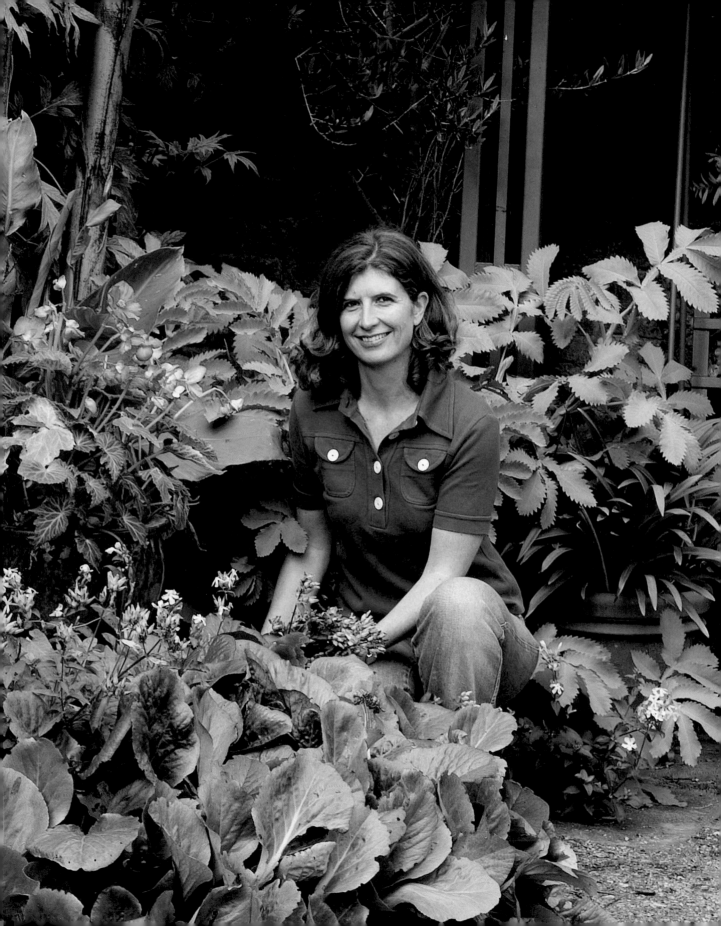

EVERY SPRING, one in twenty of the clients who walk through the door of my physiotherapy clinic is seeking help for a gardening injury. It's a staggering statistic, when you think about it: for a pastime that is meant to be pleasant and relaxing, gardening seems to cause more than its fair share of physical strife. A single session in the garden can involve bending, twisting, lifting, and kneeling, and these movements can easily throw bodies out of balance, particularly when we are unprepared for this kind of movement. Often some muscles become strong while others remain weak, and we feel sore the next day. Eventually, straining injuries can develop.

Yet my work with gardeners has been encouraging. I have found that making very small changes to their gardening technique, and showing them how to do some therapeutic, strengthening exercise before gardening and some stretching afterwards, causes many of their aches and pains to melt away—and a balanced body, deep muscle strength and good posture are welcome side effects. For gardeners, the key to improvement lies in learning to conscientiously and proactively cultivate their deep, internal muscles and a balanced body. Warming up is also important, and post-gardening stretches can go along way towards diminishing discomfort.

Though I present various exercise regimes, this is not a traditional workout manual. I won't encourage you to push yourself through hundreds of repetitions or to lift the heaviest pot you can find. Quality of movement, rather than quantity, should be your aim. The Pilates-based exercises in this chapter, which work the deep muscles, may look like very small movements—they are certainly not flashy—but they are highly rewarding. With diligent practice, looking after your body will eventually become second nature as you push your wheelbarrow, dig up weeds, and lift pots with increased strength, better posture, and reduced vulnerability to injury and strain.

Jacqueline Knox

As a physiotherapist, I enjoy
helping gardeners to build balance,
strength, coordination, and better
quality of movement.

Balancing the Body Before Gardening

Gardeners can draw particular benefit from techniques based on the Pilates method. Developed by Joseph Pilates in the early 20th century, the techniques aim to balance the body from head to toe. Pilates is often used for injury rehabilitation and is also frequently adopted by dancers. Increasingly, it is also taken up by everyday people who covet the leanness and overall feeling of balanced wellbeing it gives them.

At the heart of this body-balancing approach to fitness is the concept of building and using a strong core, which in turn equips us to stay healthy and fit while gardening. It all begins with making the effort to engage the deep stabilizing muscles, also referred to as the local muscles, which exist deep within our bodies. In contrast to global muscles, which are mobilizers and facilitate dynamic movement, the deep stabilizing muscles ground us and make us feel strong on the inside. The two systems work together in a coordinated way.

The body's core—which we can also refer to as its powerhouse—consists of the lungs, the abdominals, and the pelvis: think of them as a unit, stacked one on top of the other. If our movements stem from there—and if the core is healthy, durable, and strong—it centres our movements so that our bodies feel more balanced, and in time we become far less vulnerable to the straining and twisting injuries that gardening can cause.

Pilates-based body balancing is, in my view, a healing balm for the bad habits we pick up in daily life as we rush around, slump in chairs for hours on end, watch television to unwind, and generally put the needs of others before our own. When it comes to body balancing, practice really does yield long-lasting improvement. Many octogenarians move beautifully, largely because they grew up competing for posture badges at school. Ballet dancers find Pilates exercises very useful for the sense of core strength, balance, and poise it gives them. Even when gardeners focus on body balancing for just a fraction of the time that dancers do, they too can experience real improvement in how they move.

The exercises in this section help to correct muscle imbalances in the body as they strengthen the deep stabilizing muscles. As you practise them, you will strengthen the powerhouse of your body and build up a sort of 'corset' that surrounds your spine, front, and back. The word 'corset' is apt here—for both men and women—because when you target the stabilizing muscles you are working on your abdominal area from within. Flat and toned abdominal muscles are a welcome bonus of regular Pilates body balancing work.

THREE BASICS

The following three basics of Pilates body balancing should ideally be practised each day before you garden. They require very little in terms of time or exertion. Whatever your fitness level, familiarizing yourself with these movements and positions will help you tune in to your body.

It is best to take your time as you move through the sequence, but if you only have time to run through the movements quickly this is also worthwhile as it will essentially 'remind' your muscle memory of how it feels when your back is neither arched nor slumped, your breathing is effective, and your deep muscle system is engaged.

You will draw upon these basics throughout the book. They feature heavily in the horticultural action sequences in Chapters 4 through 6, and are also key components of the stretches described later in this chapter as well as the more aerobic 'outdoor gym' regimes detailed in Chapter 2. However, don't worry if you don't experience a palpable physical change right away. The most important part is understanding what it means to use your core muscles, to breathe properly, and to keep your spine in its neutral alignment.

You can perform these body balancing basics anywhere in the garden. If you are on a hard surface or a patio, you should use a small mat; if you do the exercises on grass, you can either lie directly on the lawn or place a blanket or towel beneath you.

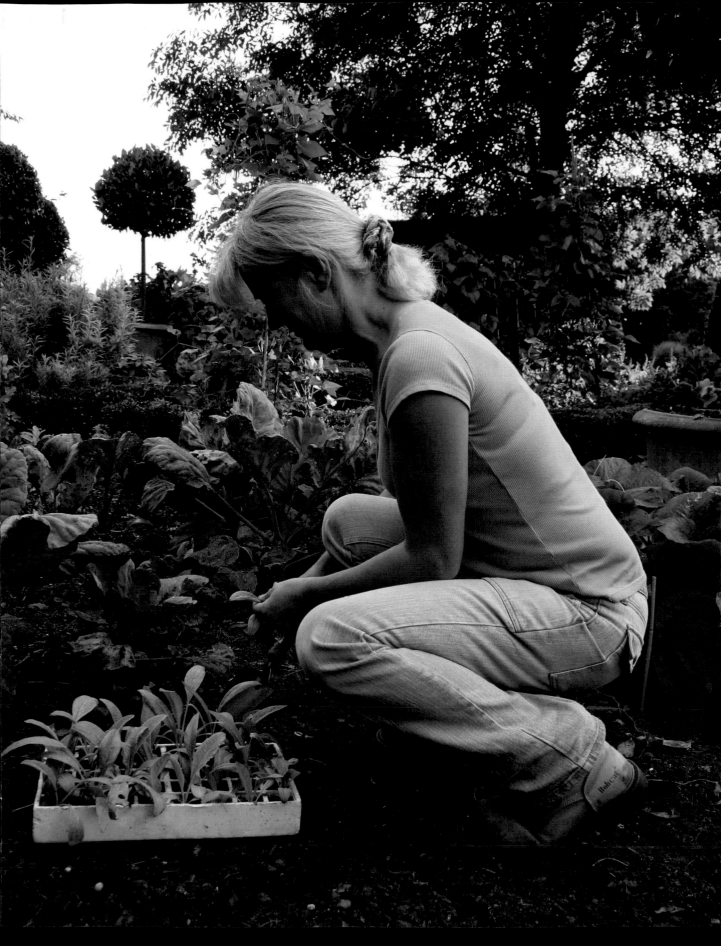

Balancing the Body Before Gardening

Finding Neutral Alignment of the Spine

Throughout this book we will refer to a neutral alignment of various parts of the body, referring to the position where least stress is placed on a given body part. To get a sense of what neutral feels like, finding neutral alignment of the spine is an excellent place to start.

Neutral alignment of the spine is halfway between your back being flattened and overarched. If you teach yourself how to find neutral before you begin gardening, you will train yourself to readily assume the neutral spine position while you are in the midst of gardening activities.

You do not need to be lying on your back or standing upright to be in neutral. Whether you are lying, standing, kneeling, sitting, or even leaning over, being in the neutral position will mean that you are neither slouching nor arching your back. Finding neutral is a small movement that may seem anticlimactic at first, but it is a highly beneficial way to prepare your body to move in a balanced manner in the garden.

• **A neutral spine retains its very subtle and natural S-shaped curves: your tailbone and ribcage should be in contact with the ground, while your pelvis is kept level and the small of your back is slightly raised.**

• **If you have a history of back pain, seek professional guidance before attempting to find neutral.**

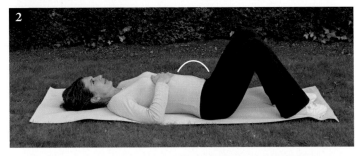

1 Lie on your back, and look down at your pelvis and the bones on either side of your pelvis; they should be level. Gently tilt your spine into the ground so that your back feels wholly flattened on the surface. As your spine imprints itself onto the ground, your pelvis will become very subtly curved.

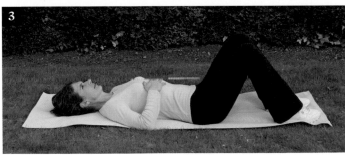

2 Then tilt your pelvis the other way so that your back is slightly arched.

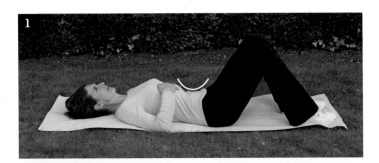

3 Finally, come back to midway between the two positions, so that your pelvis is level and your back is neither flattened into the ground nor arched: this is your spine's neutral position.

Breathing Properly

While you are lying in your neutral position, take a few minutes to practise breathing in a way that will make you feel centred. This exercise involves inhaling air into your ribcage, making maximum use of your lung capacity. The increased oxygen intake helps to rejuvenate your body, preparing you for the dynamic work you are about to undertake.

Breathe in through your nose slowly and deeply, allowing the air to gently expand your ribcage. Aim for 10–14 breaths per minute, concentrating on the feeling of being both aligned and centred. Try to breathe in neutral for at least three minutes.
- **Make the breaths deep and relaxed. Do not take huge gulps of air.**
- **Stop the exercise if you feel dizzy.**

Engaging the Deep Stabilizing Muscles

Imagine a tree with no roots blowing in the breeze; it would not take much more than a gust of wind to blow it over. Then imagine the same tree with roots that anchor it into the ground and give it a sturdy base of support. The deep stabilizing muscles of the body act like the roots of a tree; they help to support the spine and all the other joints.

The deep stabilizing muscles are also referred to as the body's powerhouse, or its centre. As you take five minutes to locate and engage these muscles before a gardening session, you are building up a strong centre from which to draw strength and balance as you reach, lift, and bend your way through the gardening session. When these deep muscles are engaged they protect and stabilize your spine as you garden. As with Finding Neutral, it is useful to concentrate on these muscles before you garden so that you can readily draw upon them when you are in the midst of a strenuous activity.

When you breathe in, lengthen your spine and neck; when exhaling, gently draw the muscles of your pelvic floor up and in, gradually incorporating your lower abdominal muscles. Your lower back itself should remain still; keep the action low, within your abdomen and below your belly button as you hollow your lower abdominal muscles back towards your spine. Start with just a few repetitions, building gradually to a sequence of 10.

- **In Pilates, this position is referred to as Four Point Kneeling.**
- **If your pelvis and spine remain completely still as you exhale, you are on the right track.**
- **Once you find these muscles in a kneeling position, you can engage them in any position. As you will see when gardening actions are detailed in later chapters, engaging these muscles is a particularly effective way to take the strain away from your back and neck.**
- **Avoid if you have any type of knee problem or hip/knee joint replacement.**
- **Do not clench or grip the stomach muscles higher up in your abdomen, as this will affect your breathing.**
- **Resist the all-too-common tendency to hold your breath while in this or any of the other body balancing positions!**

Turn onto your hands and knees, with knees beneath your hips at a right angle. Hands should be placed on the floor directly under your shoulders; elbows should be lightly bent, not locked. Your shoulder blades should be nice and stable against the chest wall. Your back should be in neutral.

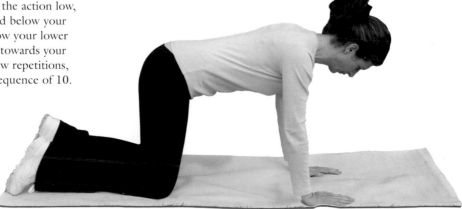

Balancing the Body Before Gardening

EIGHT PILATES EXERCISES FOR GARDENERS

Once you feel comfortable with the three basic principles of body balancing, you can move on to this series of eight Pilates exercises which have been specially chosen to benefit gardeners. When carried out before gardening, they will prepare your body for the stress it is about to experience by improving posture and stability, maintaining flexibility, and helping to prevent pulled muscles. They target the weak, deep muscles that support your spine and help to loosen the often overworked and tight muscles that bear the brunt of the strains that gardening tends to inflict.

If you have time to run through the entire set every day before gardening you should feel a real improvement in the way you carry out your daily activities, in the garden and beyond it. If you are very short on time, however, carrying out the sequence twice a week will bring about some improvement. In time you may discover that certain exercises make you feel better; as you do them, you feel pleasantly challenged and you notice a change in how you move through your gardening activities. You can then spend more time on these exercises, mixing and matching to create a bespoke workout.

Wear comfortable clothes that allow you to move easily and keep you warm. You can do these exercises on the lawn (blanket optional), or on an exercise mat placed on a paved area or a deck.

Knee Folds

Knee Folds challenge your deep muscle system. The exercise may look simple, but the goal is to keep your back in neutral and bend your knee up towards your chest without any movement or twisting in your spine or pelvic area. Your deep stabilizing muscles should be engaged.

• **To test whether you are performing Knee Folds correctly, place a ball on top of your belly button and see that it stays in position.**

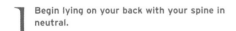

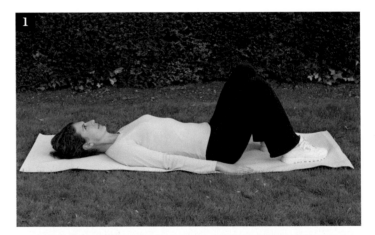

1 Begin lying on your back with your spine in neutral.

2 Bend one knee up into your chest, taking care not to flatten your spine into the floor. Lower your leg, and then repeat on the other side. Complete a series of 10 lifts.

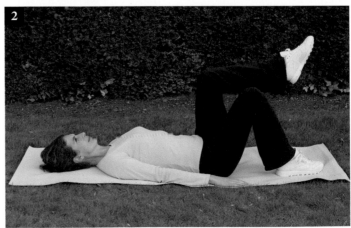

Spine Curls

For Spine Curls, begin in your neutral position: lying on your back, with knees bent up and feet on the floor. You may want to rest your head on a small pillow.

This exercise should be done slowly and with control. As you curl (and then uncurl) your spine, visualize its movement as a rolling motion that progresses vertebra by vertebra, like a wheel.

• **This is where a lawn comes in handy, as it is more comfortable for the spine to imprint itself on soft grass.**

RELEASING TENSION

Spine Curls are wonderful for lengthening your spine and moving your shoulders; the exercise will encourage movement at each individual vertebra. If you have been sitting or standing for long periods or sitting in a sustained position for hours on end, then you should feel a very satisfying stretch.

While performing this and the other exercises in this chapter, take the opportunity to centre your body and mind as you prepare for the physical activity of gardening that lies ahead. As you breathe out while gently uncurling your spine, visualize the melting away of stress and anxiety—the nagging worries that persist in your brain, and the tension that manifests itself palpably in your body, particularly in your neck and upper back. Although this is easier said than done, you should avoid tensing up during this exercise, as this can exacerbate any stiffness that you may be carrying in your back.

After a series of slow Spine Curls you should feel lengthened, relaxed, and ready for all of that reaching and pruning.

1 Once you have found neutral, breathe in and as you breathe out lift up your pelvic floor and slowly tilt your pelvis back so that you are gently imprinting the spine on the ground. As you slowly imprint your spine, your pelvis begins to tilt until your spine lifts off the ground about 3 in. (7.5 cm). Your pelvis at this point is slightly tilted backwards with your pelvic floor lifted.

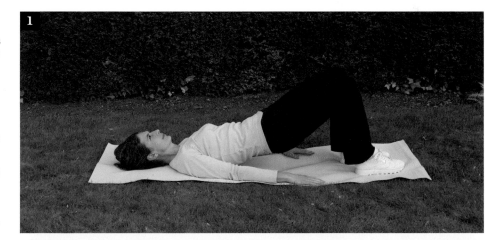

2 Then take another breath in and bring your arms up and over your head until you touch the floor behind you with the backs of your hands. Exhale while gently uncurling your spine until you are back in neutral, and then return your arms to their starting position. Do a series of 10.

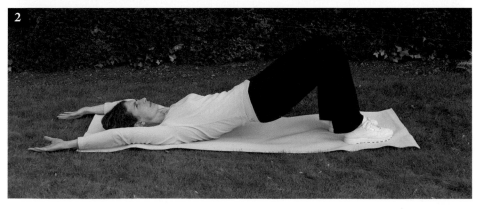

Balancing the Body Before Gardening

Side Rolls

Before beginning your Side Rolls, place a small pillow under the nape of your neck. This will help you to avoid straining your neck as it moves in a controlled manner with your head and shoulders.

This exercise will be particularly beneficial if you have been at an office hunched over a desk or in a car behind the steering wheel for hours on end. Of course, it is also beneficial for anyone prone to stooping, bending, or reaching in a way that favours one side of the body or causes discomfort in the back or the neck.

As you roll, moving your knees from their tilted position to a central neutral position and then onto the other side, it is important to take a good breath out, relieving yourself of unwanted tension in the process. The movement should feel lovely and rhythmic,

but be careful not to do it so quickly that you lose control of your deep stabilizing muscles, which should be continuously engaged; it helps to visualize the entire exercise stemming from these muscles in your lower abdomen. Remember to perform this exercise in both directions, alternating sides with each roll. Essentially this exercise teaches your body what it feels like to stay balanced and centred even while engaged in a twisting motion.

- **Draw in your deep stabilizing muscles as your knees move, being careful not to arch your back.**
- **The pillow you use should fill the hollow beneath the nape of your neck when you lie flat on the ground. Use one or two pillows depending on the size of the nape of your neck.**

1 Lie on your back in neutral position, with one arm straight out at your side to make a right angle. Inhale.

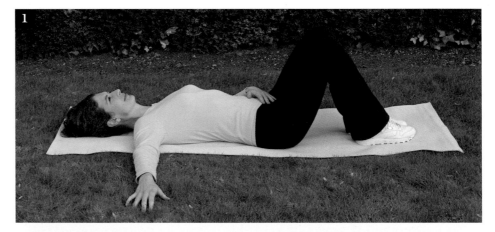

2 As you exhale, turn your head and neck towards your outstretched arm while your knees go in the other direction. Inhale and return to neutral, then exhale and turn the other way with your head and neck following your arm as your knees go the other way. Keep alternating smoothly, completing 5 rolls in each direction.

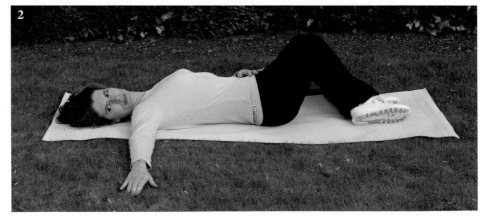

Arm Openings

Arm Openings are wonderful for gardeners as they help to mobilize a stiff upper back.
The movement is excellent preparation for the awkward twisting that gardening can entail.

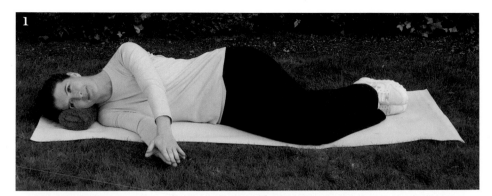

1 Begin lying on your side with pillow or rolled-up towel or sweatshirt supporting your neck. Your arms should be in front of you, with palms together. Your knees should be bent, and your spine should stay in neutral. Breathe in to prepare.

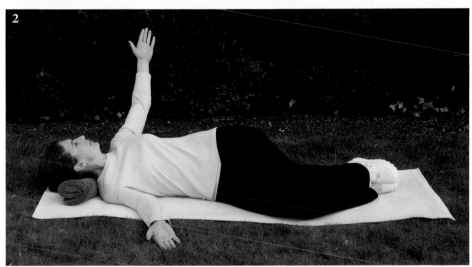

2 Exhale and open one of your arms while you rotate your thorax to that side as your arm opens out in front of you. Follow the arm's movement with your eyes. Then inhale as your upper arm returns to meet the resting arm underneath. Keep your pelvic floor and lower abdominal muscles lifted throughout. Do 5 repetitions on each side.

TWISTING IN THE GARDEN

Gardening involves many movements that cause your spine to temporarily take on a rotational position. Some of these activities, such as using a pickaxe (RIGHT), require great coordination and should not be attempted until you are comfortable with the tool you are using and feel in control of the movement.

Good technique helps to mitigate the potentially damaging nature of these activities. Arm Openings encourage movement in your upper back, and while you are in the midst of those gardening activities that cause you to twist, you should remember the feeling of moving the upper back in a healthy and well-balanced way. Engaging your core muscles throughout the movement is also beneficial.

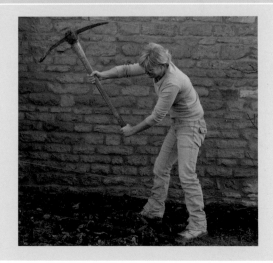

Balancing the Body Before Gardening

Diamond Press

The Diamond Press is one of those exercises that looks altogether simple, but is in fact quite challenging when carried out slowly, conscientiously, and with excellent technique.

The muscles in our backs tend to become overlooked as we cannot see them, but they are vital for keeping us upright and giving us good posture and poise. If you sit for long periods looking at a computer screen, you probably store tension in your neck, shoulders, and upper back. The Diamond Press will help to relieve some of that tension.

● **The Diamond Press produces a very small, almost invisible movement as your shoulders are lifted off of the ground while the rest of your body remains still.**

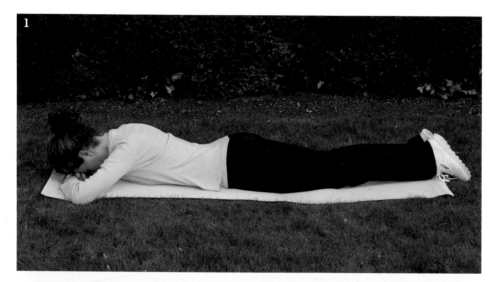

1 Begin on your stomach, with your hands under your forehead and elbows out at your sides to form a diamond shape. Your head, which rests on your hands, should be facing downwards and your legs should be straight out on the ground behind you. Inhale, feeling the air come into your lungs.

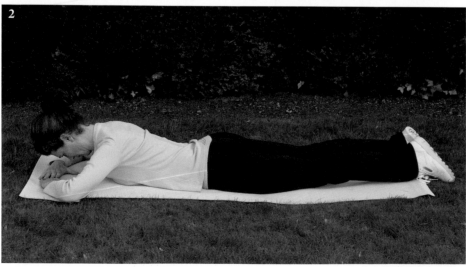

2 Then exhale, lifting your pelvic floor and slowly drawing your shoulder blades down and in towards the middle of your back. Carry out a sequence of 10.

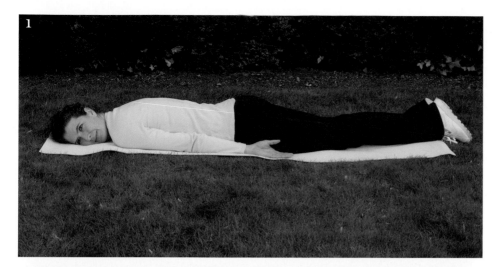

1 Begin lying on your stomach. Rest your head to one side with your arms held straight down the side of your body. Your spine should be in neutral. Inhale to prepare.

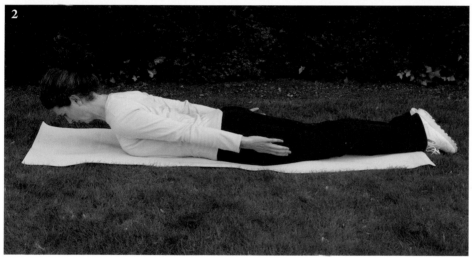

2 As you breathe out, lift up your pelvic floor and lower abdominals, drawing your shoulder blades down and in towards the centre of your back. Hold for five seconds while continuing to breathe. Slowly lower back down until you are ready to repeat. Work up to a series of 10 ten-second holds.

Dart

The Dart is an excellent exercise for working the deep muscles in your back. Here it is important not to push your stomach into the ground, and in the process to shorten your lower back. Instead, picture your back as being continuously lengthened throughout this exercise.

Performing the Dart correctly will involve having an awareness of your pelvic floor being lifted. As you lift your head and shoulders off the ground, make sure that your neck remains lengthened as if someone is pulling a string attached to the top of your head. Your spine should stay lengthened, rather than becoming compressed.

Remember to keep breathing throughout the entire exercise. Work up slowly, beginning with a series of 10 three-second holds and then working your way up to the ten-second holds.

As you lift up, you should continue looking straight down with your head, lengthening the back of your neck. You should have a sense of lengthening your entire body, all the way from your tailbone to your head.

• **Visualize your shoulder blades moving down and in on a diagonal line across to the opposite hip.**

• **If you suffer from a neck problem, dizziness, or high blood pressure, avoid turning your neck to one side; instead, just keep your face facing forwards and fold your hands under your head to cushion it.**

Balancing the Body Before Gardening

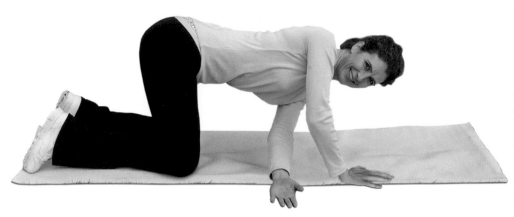

Rotation in Four Point Kneeling

Gardening involves so much twisting of the body, which can wreak havoc on the lower back. Rotation in Four Point Kneeling will train you to twist with your upper back instead, which will reduce the likelihood of injury and strain. It is also excellent for strengthening your lower abdominal muscles and building up your 'corset'. Complete 3 rotations on each side.

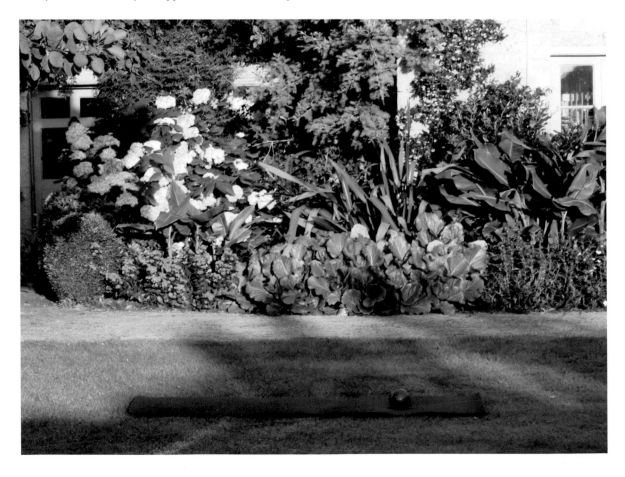

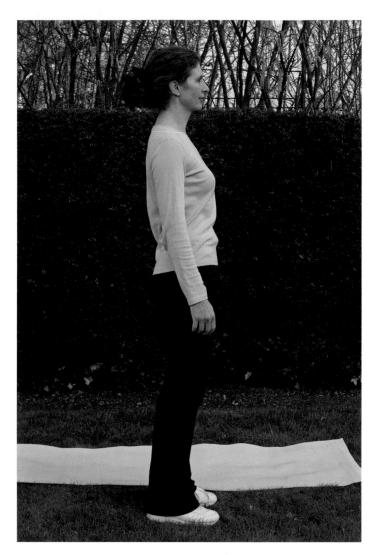

To return to neutral, stand with your feet hip-width apart, with the arches of your feet lifted. Your knees should be slightly bent, not locked, and your pelvic floor and lower stomach should be lifted. Pay attention to your back: it should be neither arched nor flattened. Your shoulder blades should be positioned down and in, towards the centre of your back. Your head should be in its neutral position: facing forward, with your chin slightly lifted.

Returning to Neutral

To finish the eight-step routine it is nice to put it all together and finish with good posture by returning to your neutral alignment of the spine in standing position.

This will give you the feeling of lengthening your body through your head, while at the same time being anchored firmly to the ground. Your foot position is important, as a neutrally positioned foot (see Chapter 3) will give you a stable base on which to stand. Try to stand on the lawn with bare feet, as feeling the grass between your toes will heighten this awareness.

IF YOU FIND THAT PILATES IS DIFFICULT...

Many people find that grasping Pilates is hard at first. It is particularly challenging if you are trying to teach yourself, so if you can find a local instructor to give you at least half a dozen initial lessons it will be time well spent. If you enjoy it, you may want to carry on and attend a weekly class to supplement exercises done at home.

If, on the other hand, you feel that Pilates is not for you, there are many alternative routines and methods that will develop your deep muscles and improve the way you move and carry yourself, both in the garden and outside of it.

For instance, the Alexander Technique, the Feldenkrais method, yoga, and tai chi, along with a range of exercise tools such as weighted balls and foam rollers (see Chapter 2) can help you to focus on the deep core postural muscles.

Exercising with a Swiss Ball (see Chapter 2) will also work your deep stabilizing muscles, balancing your body in preparation for gardening. Anything that challenges your sense of balance, such as walking on an exercise beam in your garden (see Chapter 2), will help to develop your balance and postural muscle control.

Aerobic Preparation for More Strenuous Gardening

Pilates-based body balancing targets your deep muscles and sets you up to carry out gardening tasks in a more balanced way, and on its own it is often adequate preparation for moderate gardening activity. However, if you are embarking on a session of strenuous gardening—which can be defined as anything that will make you break a sweat—you should carry out some additional aerobic warmup exercise first. This aerobic preparation should last from 10 to 15 minutes, and the only criterion is that you should be continuously moving about. If you find yourself feeling physically warmer, this means you are doing it effectively.

WHY WARM UP?

Warming up literally gets your blood flowing, and with increased blood flow to your muscles, the muscles' temperature increases. Once your muscles have been 'woken up' and set in motion, they become increasingly coordinated as you repeat the exercise. This increased coordination helps to protect you from injury and strain.

On an emotional level, warming up serves the important purpose of getting you 'in the mood' to be active. Just as athletes use their warmup sessions to mentally prepare for competition, warming up before gardening prepares your brain to tell your muscles to get ready for the work ahead.

Take a brisk walk around the garden, go up and down some steps, or march up and down the patio—anything to get moving and warm. As you warm up, take the opportunity to look around; survey what needs to be done in the garden, and contemplate how you will accomplish your goals. Take time to admire the plants that are flourishing and the fruits and vegetables that are doing well, and enjoy the space, fresh air, and birdsong.

You can even warm up while sipping a cup of coffee or tea, because the warmup should never make you feel like you are overexerting yourself. If you have the tendency to get out of breath easily, start out by doing only what feels comfortable (even if this is just five minutes of steady walking about the garden), and build up slowly as your stamina increases. Your heart rate should not be too high during the session; you should be able to comfortably hold a conversation during the warmup.

If it is cold outside, you might need to wear an extra layer such as a fleece or a sweatshirt while you warm up. It is important to keep warm as you gradually increase your heart rate through activity. Once you feel that you are warm and ready for a session of strenuous gardening or exercise, then you can shed the extra layer.

After you have warmed up and are ready to embark on your gardening tasks, pace yourself: start slowly and work up to the more demanding actions such as marathon weeding sessions or long periods pushing a heavy mower. As you carry out more strenuous gardening it is important that you limit periods of intensive labour so that you do a small amount of gardening regularly, rather than long spurts of gardening once in a rare while.

Moreover, you should regularly change jobs so that different muscle groups are used; do not, for instance, prune tree branches high above your head for more than a half hour at a time. If you suffer from back or joint pain then you need to take extra care by stopping what you are doing and moving on to a new activity as soon as your problem areas feel any strain.

ONE SAMPLE WARMUP
• *Brisk walking* (see page 46): 4 minutes
• *Lunges* (see page 47): 4 minutes
• *Step-ups* (see page 48): 2 minutes

A brisk walk down this garden path will warm you up in preparation for a strenuous gardening session.

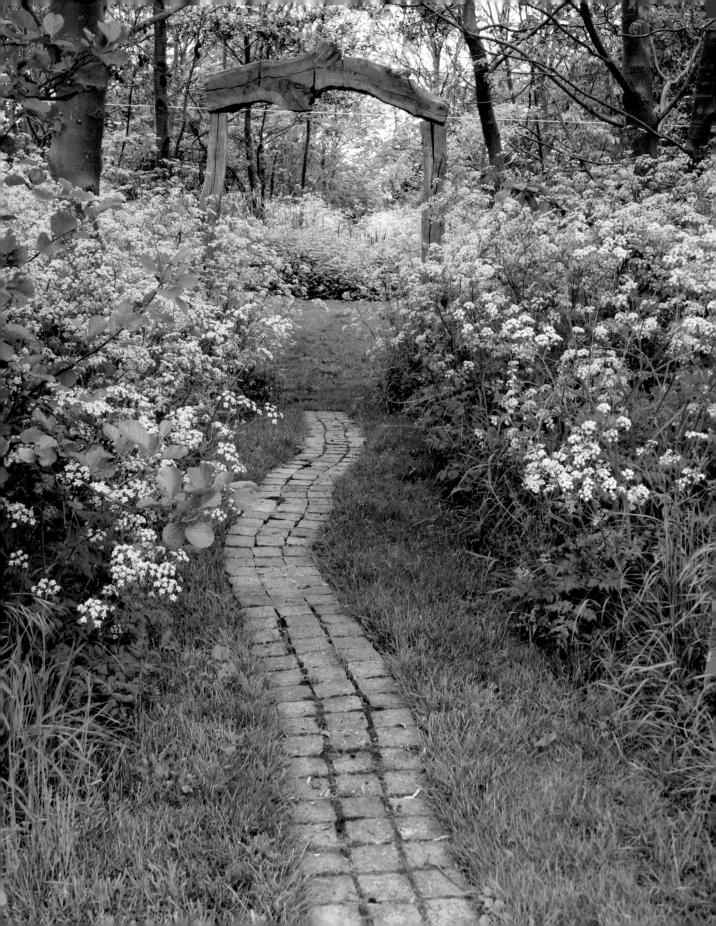

Post-Gardening Stretches

Many gardeners complain of stiffness after a day spent gardening. This stiffness is more likely to occur if they have taken on too much in the garden when their muscles are unaccustomed to working hard.

Stretching is an important part of treating your muscles well and protecting them from injury; it can significantly lessen the post-exercise stiffness that tends to afflict so many of us. If you take the time to stretch after a gardening session, you will find that your muscles 'complain' far less during the days that follow.

Stretching works by lengthening muscles and reducing tightness in them. Because muscles are composed of tissue that is elastic, they are prone to being lengthened, but also to tightening up. After physical activity or exertion muscles adapt to the stress of the exercise by shortening, so it makes sense to stretch after a bout of exercise when the muscles are nicely warmed up and more pliable.

If you stretch regularly, you should experience a change in the way that you move. Take the leg lengthening stretch, for instance: after repeating this regularly for a few weeks, you will find that you can bend with far more ease when you reach down to grab hold of a weed or to pick up a plant. Greater strength can be achieved by simply remaining in the stretching positions for longer. To become more flexible, try to push your muscles to stretch a bit further each time. On the other hand, however, it is absolutely vital to listen to your body and never force a stretch when it feels uncomfortable.

The Best Stretches for Gardeners

There are so many ways to stretch, and they all seem to go in and out of fashion. The following stretches have been chosen to counteract common gardeners' problems such as stiffness in the lower back and tightness in the hamstrings. They are absolutely essential when you have been doing something involving leaning over or kneeling for long periods, such as weeding. Although you will feel the impact of the stretches, they should not be painful—so be sure to stop the stretch if you feel any pain.

If you don't have time to do the entire series, you can hand-pick the ones that stretch any muscles that feel particularly tight. Each stretch should be sustained for 30 to 60 seconds and carried out a total of 6 times, with 3 stretches on each side.

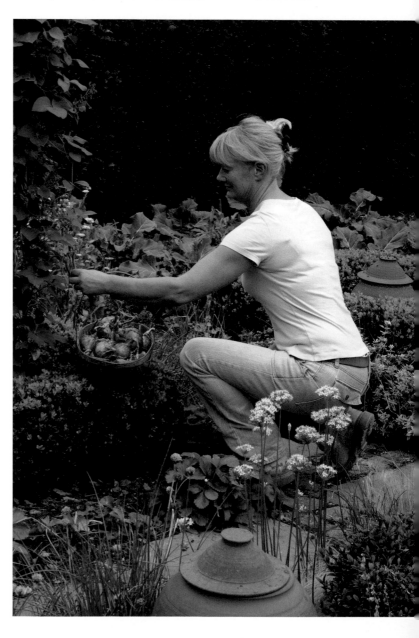

Regular stretching improves movement, enabling you to perform actions like squatting to pick beans with greater ease.

GUIDELINES FOR STRETCHING SAFELY

1 Avoid stretching before you begin moving in the garden—but always stretch afterwards. Stretching before you warm up or begin working in the garden will mean you are stretching cold muscles, which can be dangerous. Imagine your muscle system as a ball of clay that is cold and hard to mould at first; once you warm it up, it becomes more malleable. If you stretch while your muscles are cold, you risk a straining injury. Stretching before gardening is a common gardeners' pitfall, and a major cause of injury.

2 Don't push yourself to stretch too far before you are ready to do so—and never force a stretch. A muscle should not be forced into a range of movement until it is strong and comfortable in that range.

3 When you stretch, it is important to think about your posture at the same time. For example when you stretch your hamstrings make sure that your back stays in neutral. This way the stretch occurs in your leg, rather than your back.

4 Stretch slowly. Sudden jerky movements or violent stretching must be avoided. The body has its inbuilt protective mechanisms, and if you overstretch too violently the stretch reflex in the your muscle is activated and the muscle actually responds by tightening up so that you become stiffer. This response is due to your nervous system protecting your muscles from damage.

5 Finally, make sure you keep breathing throughout your stretching session.

Leg Lengthening

With Leg Lengthening, the key is to keep your lumbar (lower) spine in neutral. Do not lock your knees. The stretch will be felt in your hamstrings. You may want to use a band or scarf to help you stretch, although lightly gripping your thigh with your hands is just as effective. Your back must stay in neutral as you stretch; if you find yourself arching your back, you are stretching too far. Lift your pelvic floor muscles throughout the stretch.

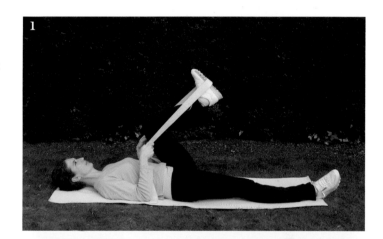

1 Lie on your back and bring your knee towards your chest.

2 Then attempt to straighten this leg as much as possible, feeling the stretch in the back of your upper thigh.

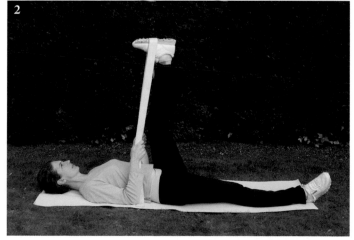

Post-Gardening Stretches

Hip Loosening

Hip Loosening will target your gluteal muscles, helping to alleviate tension around the lower back. Keep your pelvic floor muscles lifted, and your back in neutral throughout the stretch; in order to do so, you will need to engage your core muscles. Skip if you have knee problems.

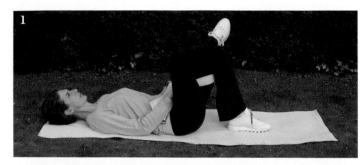

1 Bend one knee into your chest and hook the foot of the other leg over the knee of the bent-up leg.

2 Slowly pull the bent leg towards your chest without losing neutral or twisting your back or neck.

Thigh Stretch

This is an excellent stretch that targets your hip flexors and groin. You can do it while lying down, standing up, or—unless you have any knee problems—in a kneeling position. Lift your pelvic floor throughout.

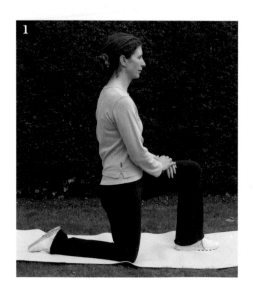

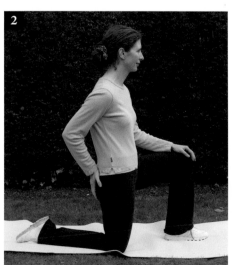

1 Begin with your back in neutral. Place one leg out in front of you, bent at roughly a right angle.

2 Place one hand on your bottom and push gently forwards until you feel a stretch at the front of your thigh and groin area.

1 Kneeling with your back in neutral and with one knee bent in front of you, bring one arm up and out to the side and then over your head.

2 Lean to the side in the direction of your supporting leg, keeping your lower abdominals lifted, before returning to the centre.

Side Stretch

Side Stretch targets the latissimus dorsi muscles on the sides of your body. It should be felt just under your armpit and down

into your chest. The challenge here is to keep your torso facing forwards; although you are leaning, you are not twisting. Skip this one if you have shoulder problems.

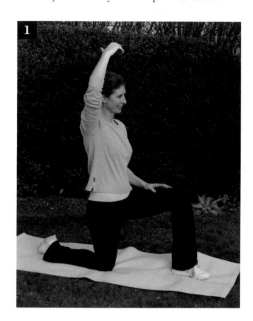

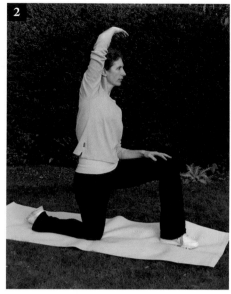

1 Standing in neutral, bend one arm inwards at about a right angle. Then lightly grasp this elbow with the hand of your other arm.

2 Keeping your arms in this position, bring them slowly up in front of your body as far as you can without arching your back. Then gently pull on your elbow until you feel the stretch. Bring your arms down in front of your body. Switch your arms before repeating.

Upper Arm Stretch

This stretch targets your triceps. Do not tilt your head up when your arms are over your head; keep looking straight ahead

throughout the stretch. Remember to continue grasping your elbow as you move your arms in front of your body. Your pelvic floor and lower abdominals should be lifted.

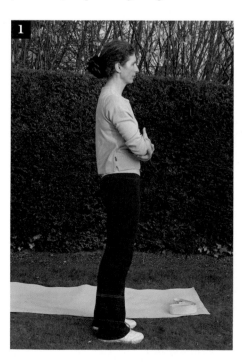

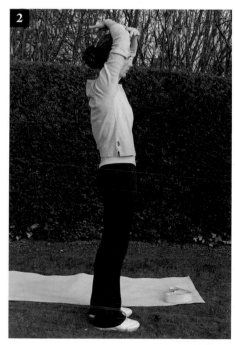

Post-Gardening Stretches

STRETCHING AND STRENGTHENING: FINDING YOUR BALANCE

It is unwise to focus on stretching without also focusing on building up strength. The reason for this is simple: if you improve your flexibility and have a large range of movement without also having the strength to control this movement, then you become vulnerable to strain. Conversely, if you are very strong but lack have the flexibility to carry out a certain movement, then you run the risk of strain as well. A sound solution lies in combining strength with flexibility. Ideally, you should aim not only to be flexible enough to get into a given Pilates position, but also strong enough to be able to hold it; it is, yet again, a matter of aiming for a good balance.

Because we are all individuals with different needs, it is vital that we hone in on our strengths and weaknesses as we equip ourselves to garden in a safe and healthy way. Some of us are flexibile and can be too mobile, while others tend towards being stiff and inflexible. Some of us are naturally strong, or find it relatively easy to build up muscle strength, while others have always found it very difficult to lift heavy things. While we should aim for a balance between stretching and strengthening, if you feel you are particularly weak in one area or the other then you should focus on those exercises that seem to bring about improvement. If you are prone to certain symptoms such as a stiff upper back or tight shoulders, make an effort to exercise in a way that will address those needs (see below).

Our minds are so closely linked to our bodies. When we are stressed or anxious we tend to stiffen up, and at other times we relax by collapsing and becoming soft and flexible. Our minds control the way we move, and our nervous systems adapt to the demands that are placed on our bodies. In this sense, cultivating our emotional health is an essential element of fitness that should never be overlooked.

Stretching up towards the sky with a stable base and a strong centre while looking at a stunning view can be highly invigorating.

PERSONALIZING YOUR WORKOUT

Although we are all different, certain stresses, strains, and injuries seem to be very prevalent among gardeners. Techniques for counteracting specific maladies are explored in more detail in Chapter 3—but it can also be very beneficial to build your own routine of pre-gardening body balancing and post-gardening stretches so that your individual needs are addressed. Gardeners who tend to experience the following conditions may find the following exercises especially helpful.

• Tight hamstrings: Leg Lengthening (page 31)

• Stiffness in the hip area: Hip Loosening and Thigh Stretch (page 32)

• Tight shoulders: Side Rolls (page 22) and Upper Arm Stretch (page 33)

• Stiffness in the upper back: Arm Openings (page 23), Side Rolls (page 22), and Spine Curls (page 21)

• Stiffness in the neck: Side Rolls (page 22) and Diamond Press (page 24)

• A weak centre: Finding Neutral Alignment of the Spine (page 18), Engaging the Deep Stabilizing Muscles (page 19), Spine Curls (page 21), and Knee Folds (page 20)

Although a suggested number of repetitions is given alongside the step-by-step exercises earlier in this chapter, it is important to understand that these are only guidelines. They are not meant to be prescriptive; instead, they should be seen as a jumping-off point for creating a health programme that really improves the way you move through the garden (as well as the rest of your life). Instead of following the previously described regime religiously, it can be immensely rewarding to listen to what your body is telling you—and to adjust your workout accordingly.

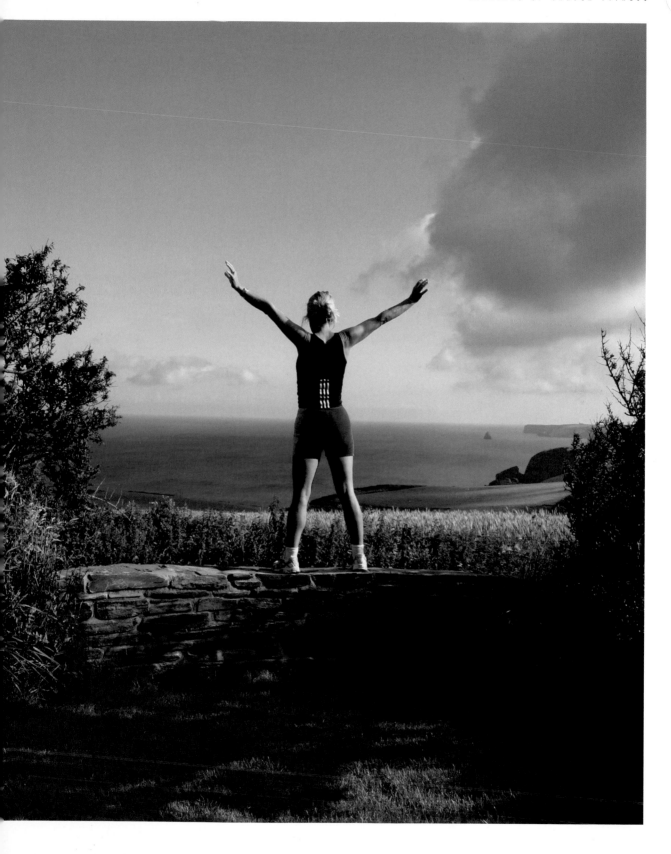

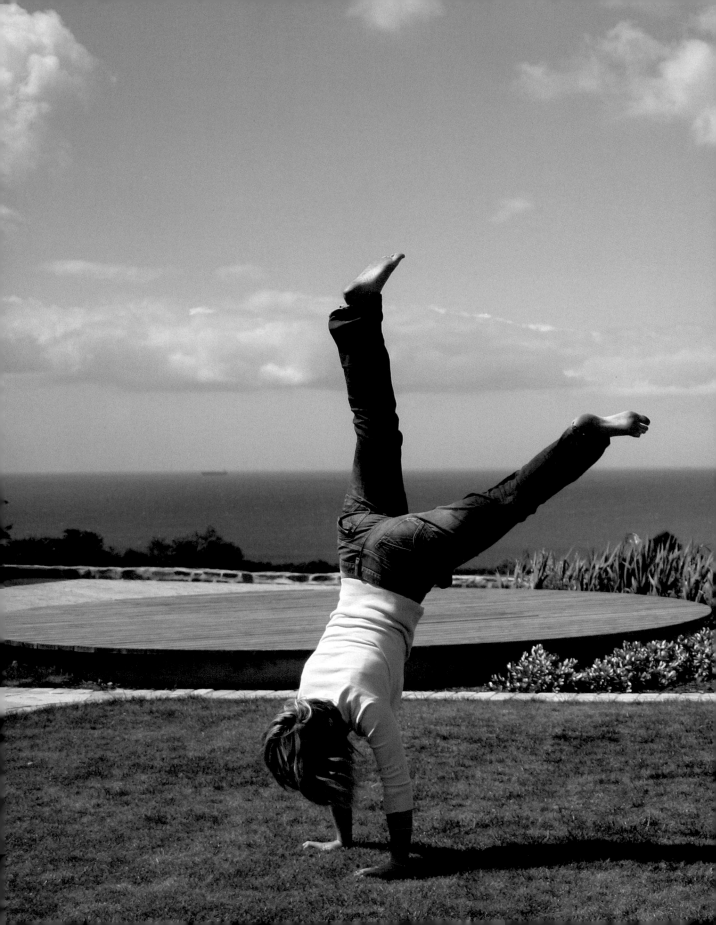

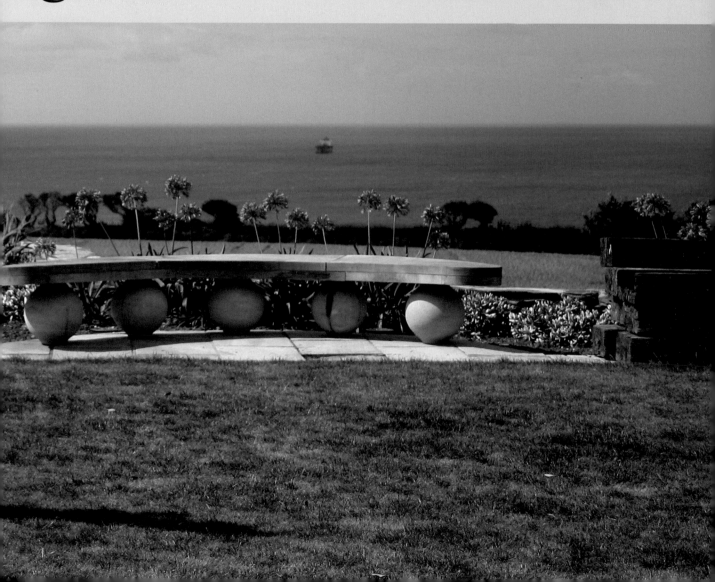

CHAPTER 2

USING YOUR OUTDOOR GYM

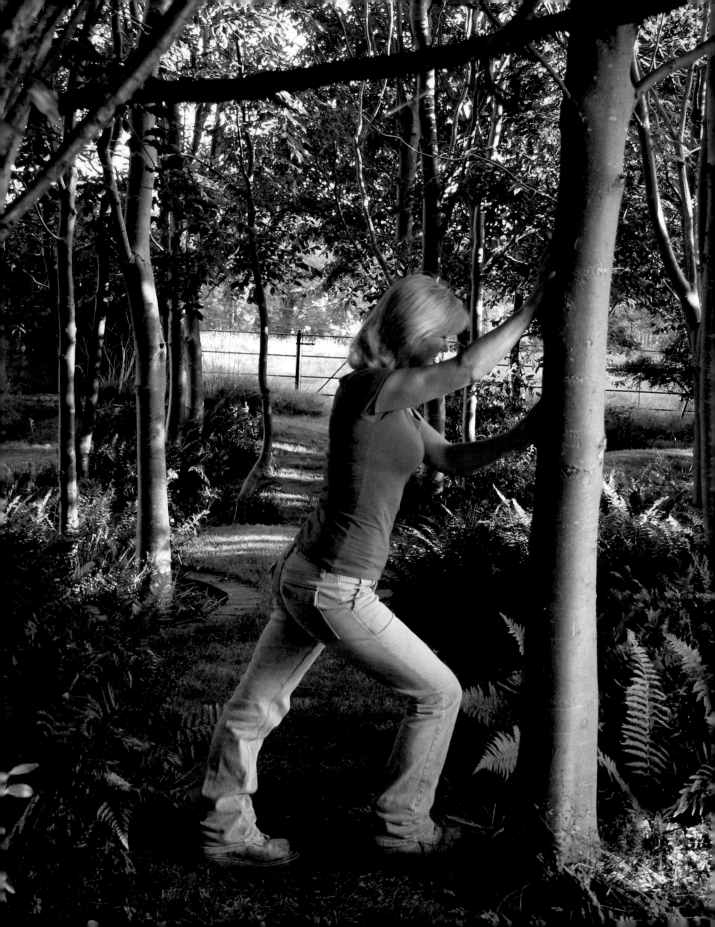

THERE ARE not many forms of exercise that we normally carry out happily for prolonged periods of time. An hour on an exercise machine at the gym often involves another half hour commuting there and back, and when it uses up your precious free time the whole routine can feel like a chore. For many of us, however, spending hours in the garden—cultivating a patch of personal space, designing it to fit our needs, and planting in the fresh air—is sheer bliss, and when we work in the garden, the minutes and hours seem to fly by. A long period spent in the garden will burn an impressive amount of calories; as the chart on the next page shows, an hour spent weeding burns around 290 calories.

To enhance your fitness level further still and burn even more calories, you can carry out some additional exercise in the garden. This may take the form of an aerobic exercise routine, a session using a Swiss Ball, or some balancing exercises using a homemade trim trail in a shady woodland clearing. Exercise regimes that are practised outdoors in the midst of the sights, sounds, and textures of your garden are rarely boring and will more than likely inspire you to continue with your workout regimes so that you experience improvement over time. At the end of an outdoor exercise session, it is nice to wind down by breathing deeply in your favourite part of the garden.

In many ways, the garden—where you are most relaxed—is an ideal place for cultivating the health of your body and mind. In this chapter, we will explore how to get the most out of your outdoor workout. Whether you are are jogging down a garden path, doing resistance exercise like squats, or turning compost, having good technique will equip you to reap as much fitness benefit as possible from the time you spend being active in your garden.

Taking some time out of a dynamic gardening session to perform a calf stretch against a nearby tree is a satisfying feeling.

Burning Calories Through Gardening

As you carry out the planting and maintenance actions that make up your gardening routine, you use your body in a wide range of positions incorporating various muscle groups and burn calories in the process. Crucially, you can use your garden's maintenance demands to motivate you and keep you on track.

Many aspects of gardening are perceived as 'gentle' exercise, but the calories that you will burn are often surprising high. Lying down, you use only about 2% of possible calorific expenditure, while sitting is marginally higher at 4% and standing around uses about 12%. However, when you bend down to remove weeds from a border, your calorific expenditure jumps up to about 35%. In the chart on the right you can see just how much your calorific expenditure increases when you, for instance, start bending to weed compared to watching television.

In our busy lives, it certainly makes sense to incorporate exercise into our daily routine, be it walking the children to school or spending half an hour in the garden before work. Spades and plants can replace the dumbbells and treadmills. Gardening lets you benefit from fresh air and (with luck) sunshine as you work out your body.

By gardening you achieve a goal as well as benefiting from being outside. Non-stop gardening can burn about 2 calories per pound per hour, which amounts to 280 calories for someone weighing 140 pounds (10 stone). The chart on the right shows the approximate number of calories various gardening actions burn, and how these compare to doing office work, driving in a car or just sitting on the sofa. (Adapted from R. J. Maughan's *Nutrition in Sport*; for more details on calorific expenditure for various body weights, see the Appendix.)

Chapters 4 to 6 contain instructions for carrying out many of these gardening activities in the healthiest possible way. Meanwhile, if you want to burn even more calories and increase your physical fitness, you can us the garden as a space for performing outdoor exercise regimes.

GARDENING CALORIE CHART

Activity	Calories burned per hour
(Approximate values based on a 140-pound person)	
Sitting watching television	60
Light office work	90
Driving fast	125
Carrying heavy loads, e.g. large pots	510
Carrying, loading, or stacking wood	325
Carrying logs	710
Chopping logs with axe, fast-paced	1,100
Chopping logs with axe, slow-paced	325
Chopping wood, splitting logs	385
Clearing land, hauling branches	325
Collecting grass or leaves	260
Digging, spading, filling garden	325
Gardening with heavy power tool, tilling a garden	385
Laying turf or crushed rock	325
Planting seedlings or shrubs	260
Planting trees	295
Raking lawn	260
Spreading soil with shovel	325
Trimming shrubs or trees with power trimmers	234
Trimming shrubs or trees with shears (secateurs)	290
Walking, applying fertilizer or seeding a lawn	155
Watering lawn or garden	90
Weeding	290

RIGHT: **Digging burns about 325 calories per hour for a 140-pound person.**

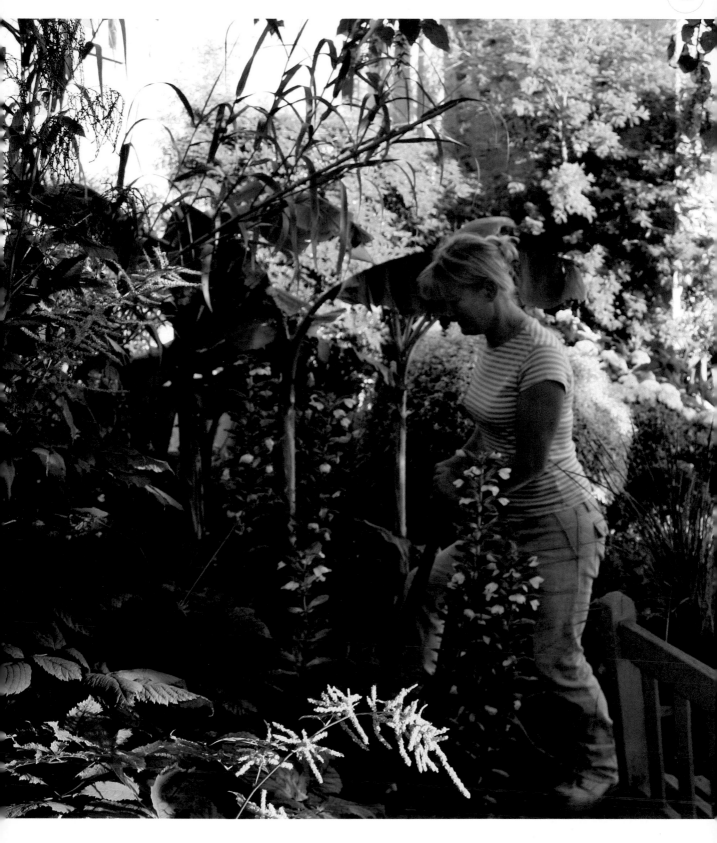

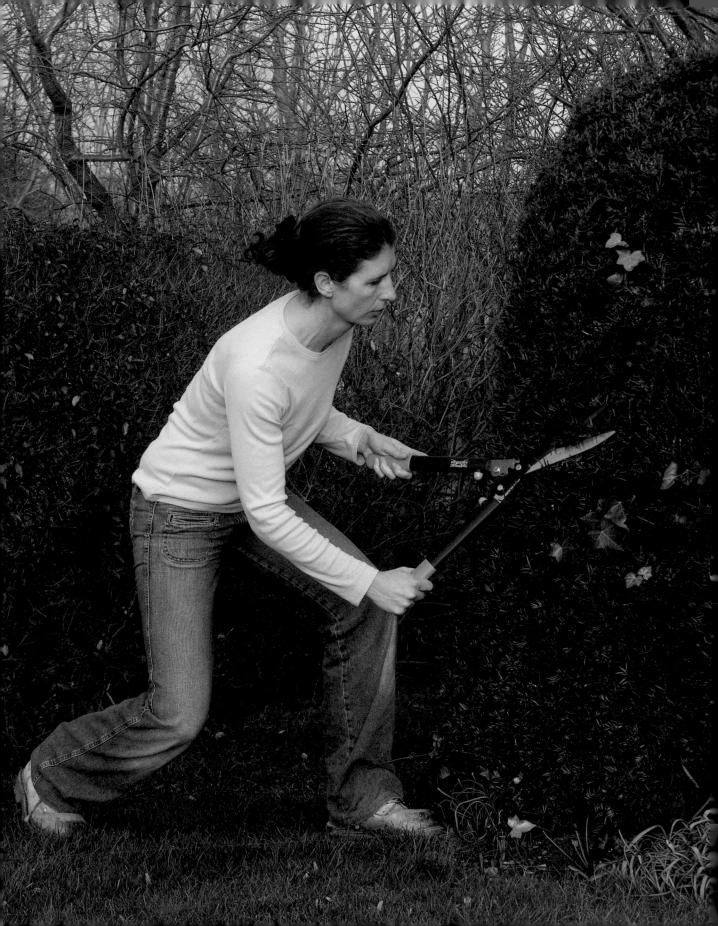

HEART RATE TRAINING ZONES

Being active in the garden and burning calories will affect your heart rate. It is useful to be aware of your heart rate when gardening, partly so that you do not overdo it and also to use it as a tool to get fitter. If your heart rate is too low you might not be working your heart and lungs effectively enough, while you will become exhausted very quickly if it is too high. Ideally you should aim to work at between 65% and 85% of your maximum heart rate, whether you are being active in the garden or carrying out an aerobic workout.

To calculate your maximum heart rate (MHR), use the Karvonen formula: MHR = 220 minus your age. If you are 40 years old, then, your MHR is 180 beats per minute. (If you are particularly unfit or have not done any exercise for a long while, subtract 20 again to reach 160 beats/minute.) Do not exceed your maximum heart rate.

SAFETY FIRST

To stay safe during exercise sessions, remember the following:

- When exercising, pace yourself gradually.

- If you feel dizzy, faint, or very short of breath, stop immediately and seek medical advice.

- Never exercise having just eaten; allow 2 hours before doing so.

- Remain hydrated and wear a sunhat if appropriate.

- Stop if you feel pain.

- Change position regularly.

- Exercise places strain on the body and this is contraindicated in certain medical conditions. To be safe, always get a medical checkup first.

- Finally: never plunge into an intensive exercise session if your body isn't ready. By regularly gardening or working out for significant periods of time, you will increase your endurance steadily.

Your upper training zone limit is 85% of your maximum heart rate, so for a 40-year-old it would be $180 \times 0.85 = 153$. This 40-year-old's lower training zone limit is 65% of their maximum heart rate: $180 \times 0.65 = 117$. Their training zone would then be between 117 and 153 beats per minute. Working at this rate, their heart would be benefiting from this exercise.

Most gardening falls into the category of endurance exercise, which means that you work out for a longer period at a lower heart rate (in the case above, this would be 117 beats per minute, or 65% of the MHR). Regular, sustained gardening—which might involve mowing the lawn, planting, or weeding—is likely to improve your endurance fitness.

Ideally, you should be combining endurance exercise with some resistance work such as turning compost which will typically bring your heart rate up to 85% of its maximum. Heavier gardening tasks, such as fast raking or shovelling, will also make your heart work at a rate nearer to its upper training level (153 beats per minute, or 85% of the MHR).

The aerobic workouts described in the next session would also bring you closer to your upper training level. Although it is excellent for burning calories, this kind of exercise would only be sustainable for shorter periods of time—unless, of course, you are already very fit.

Taking Your Pulse

The pulse can be taken in the wrist, in the neck or in the face. In the neck the pulse is quite strong and can be the easiest to feel: if you follow the edge of the jaw down about an inch into the neck, you will feel a pulsation just in front of the neck muscle. Always take the pulse with your index finger and middle finger, rather than your thumb. Count the number of beats per minute, or alternatively you can count for fifteen seconds and multiply this by four to get the number of beats per minute.

You might consider buying a heart rate monitor as they are inexpensive and very useful. If you wear one while you are exercising and gardening you will quickly and easily become aware of your different levels of exertion while doing different activities.

LEFT: Trimming hedges can involve using the entire body in a dynamic way. Exercising in the garden develops the balance, coordination, and posture you draw upon while performing actions like this.

Outdoor Dynamic Workouts

As a supplement to your gardening sessions, you can burn even more calories and build up your endurance levels by doing a series of dynamic exercises in the garden. Think of the garden as a true outdoor gym; you can do lunges in a grassy area in a woodland clearing, walk up and down steps, and jog down a garden path—the possibilities are limitless. It is satisfying to think that you can tailor your garden to accommodate— and in fact, encourage—your fitness work. (For more on this, see Chapters 4 to 6.)

Traditional gym-based routines can be boring; many of us need some sort of stimulation (whether visual, auditory, or simply filled with things that have meaning to us) in order to become absorbed in the exercise. Performing fitness routines outdoors, in a space that we have had a hand in creating, brings enhanced sensory awareness into the equation. When we exercise outdoors we start to appreciate the intricacies of our surroundings, such as the smell of lavender or the spectacle of birds having a bath. Instead of rushing around frantically, we are literally taking time to smell the roses (and exercise among them).

The Surgeon General (in the United States) recommends that we carry out about half an hour of aerobic exercise five times a week—and many fitness professionals suggest doing more. A recognized recommendation is to do 10,000 steps a day. (Try wearing a step counter during a gardening day, or a day when you exercise outside, and compare it to a 'non-gardening' day—you should notice a difference!)

RIGHT: A paved area in the middle of an elaborate planting scheme would be a great spot for practising lunges, squats, and step-ups.

BELOW: This garden path is an inviting space for brisk walking or jogging.

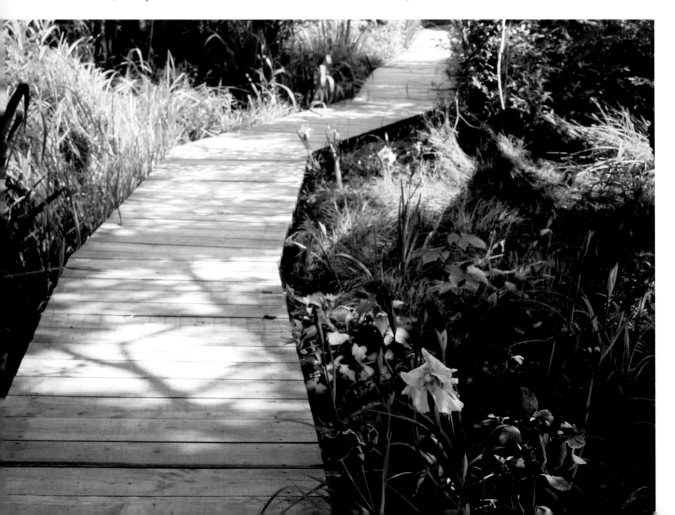

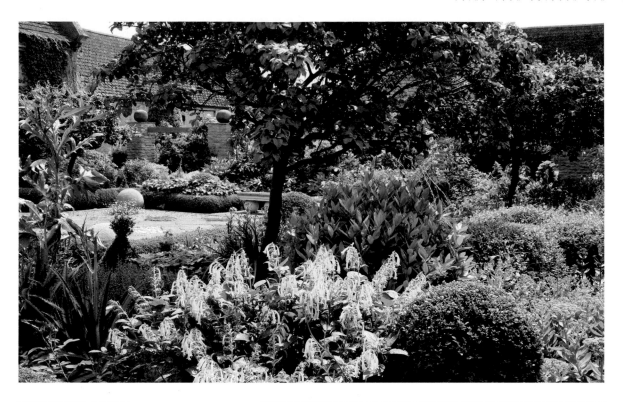

WORKOUT MENU

If you enjoy the challenge of building up your fitness levels over time, you can follow the sequence of your choice on the right.

In order to see a tangible improvement in your level of physical fitness and endurance, try to run through your chosen sequence two or three times each week and then advance to the next level as you gain in confidence. For instance, you might start with two 'easy' workouts per week and then work your way up to three 'moderate' workouts as your fitness levels improve over time. (Of course, if you are seasoned gym-goer or an athlete you will want to begin at a higher level.)

Easy workouts that are performed with great technique and attention to detail carry much more benefit than more difficult workouts that are performed carelessly or incorrectly. If you think about your alignment, deep muscle control, and proper breathing as well as concentrating on your technique, the workout becomes one of quality rather than just quantity; instead of rushing through your workout, it really pays dividends if you carry it out slowly and focus on how you are performing the movements.

THREE OUTDOOR EXERCISE REGIMES

Easy	Moderate	Advanced
Walking		
5 minutes	8 minutes	10 minutes
Running		
5 minutes	8 minutes	10 minutes
Squats		
8 repetitions	10 repetitions	15 repetitions
Lunges		
8 on each leg	10 on each leg	15 on each leg
Step-ups		
2 minutes	3 minutes	4 minutes
Skipping		
1 minute	1.5 minutes	2 minutes
Back extensions		
8 repetitions	10 repetitions	15 repetitions
Abdominal curls		
5 normal curls	6 oblique curls	20 oblique curls
	15 normal curls	5 reverse curls

Outdoor Dynamic Workouts

WORKOUT ELEMENTS

As with the gardening actions (discussed throughout Chapters 4–6), it is important to carry out the elements of the workouts in a way that keeps your body balanced, decreases your vulnerability to injury, and optimizes fitness benefits so you can get the most out of the workout.

Walking

Walking is a fabulous way to keep fit as you can do it anywhere. It is essential to have the right footwear—choose supportive trainers (sneakers) or boots that support your foot in a neutral position and do not rub the back of your heel or tendon (see Chapter 3). The lawn offers a nice spongy walking surface, while a patio, deck, or gravel area will provide you with a harder surface if you want to feel more stable.

Posture is key to good walking, so keep your back in neutral. Your lower abdominals should be lifted up and in to support your lower back. Set your shoulder blades down towards the centre of your back and keep your neck long and relaxed, with your head upright and looking forwards. Keep your arms close to your body as you move them, alternating with your legs. Your bottom muscles (gluteals) provide the push-off for each step and propel you forwards.

Forty-five minutes of walking is good aerobic exercise in itself. It is especially beneficial when carried out steadily over time; three 45-minute sessions of brisk walking per week is great exercise.

Running

As with walking, you should maintain an upright posture while running, with your lower abdominals lifted and your back held in neutral. Your arms will provide momentum. Keep them relaxed but close to your body. Do not allow your shoulders to creep up towards your ears when you start to get tired. With every step, your heel should hit the ground as you roll through your whole foot.

As you run, lift your lower abdominal muscles and stay as upright as possible. This path is made of Indian stone pieces with manmade 'ammonite' laid between them to achieve a dynamic, curved line.

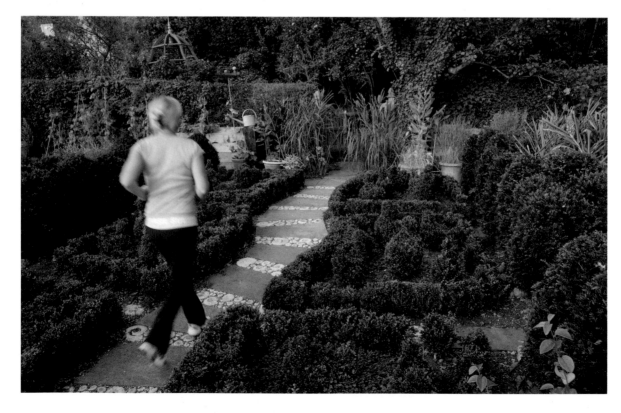

Squats

Squats are excellent for working the thigh and gluteal muscles. Keep your head lifted and your back neutral throughout even as your torso naturally leans forwards. Do not rush through the movement.

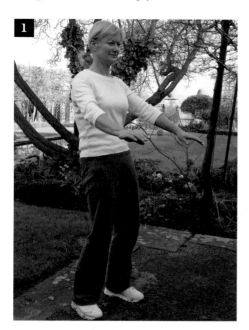

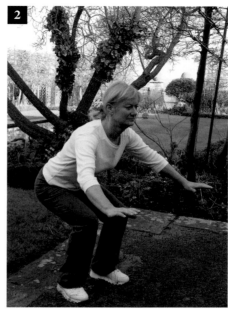

1 Stand with your feet hip-width apart, with kneecaps positioned above the second toe. Make sure that you do not rotate either of your legs inward.

2 Keep your heels on the ground (unless your calves feel uncomfortably tight, in which case you can lift them slightly). Bend your knees to slightly less than a right angle. Then return to standing and repeat.

Lunges

Lunges are great for giving a workout to your thighs and buttocks. Make sure that you complete the lunge on both sides to balance your body. Challenge yourself to keep your back straight as your body lowers.

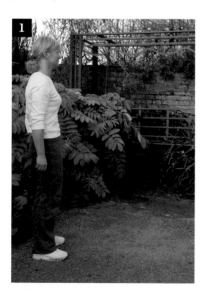

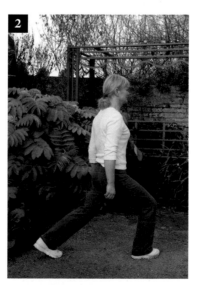

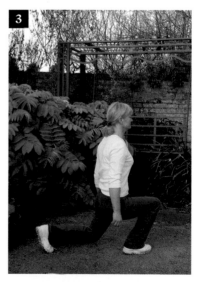

1 Begin standing up straight with your back in neutral.

2 Place one foot forward about one stride length, shifting your weight onto the front leg. Bend your knees so that the knee is in alignment with the foot, and then transfer your weight onto the front leg.

3 Bend your front leg and keep your back straight as you gradually lower yourself down. Then return to starting position and repeat.

Outdoor Dynamic Workouts

Step-ups

Step-ups tone your bottom. If done at a quicker pace, they also offer some aerobic exercise.

You can use almost any stable surface in your garden as a step—as long as it is high enough to give you a decent workout, but not so high that it is a struggle for you to step onto.

Doing 100 step-ups on each leg will give you a serious aerobic workout. This is an advanced option, though, so you should start with fewer repetitions and build up slowly.

Remember to switch to a different starting leg halfway through the routine. Keep your lower abdominals lifted throughout to enhance the workout.

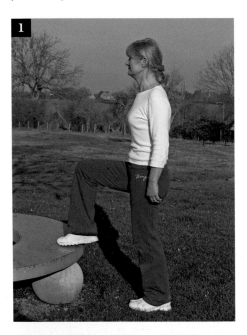

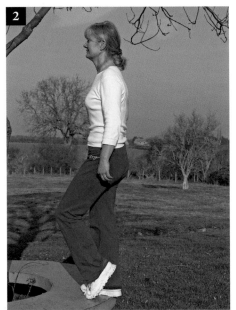

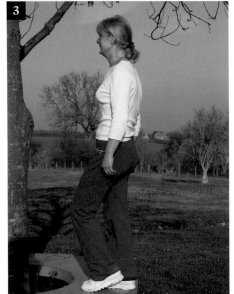

1 Stand with your right leg resting on the step in front of you. Your back should be in neutral.

2 Maintain an upright posture as you step up with your left leg.

3 Lower your left leg onto the step and transfer your weight onto your right leg before stepping down with your right leg, followed by your left leg. Repeat.

Skipping

Skipping with a rope is hard aerobic exercise and an effective calorie burner. Initially you might only be able to do it for a minute without stopping.

Build up gradually so that you do not get too breathless and skip with alternate legs so that it is not too jarring on your knees. Get into a nice rhythm as you work your way up to five minutes of continuous skipping.

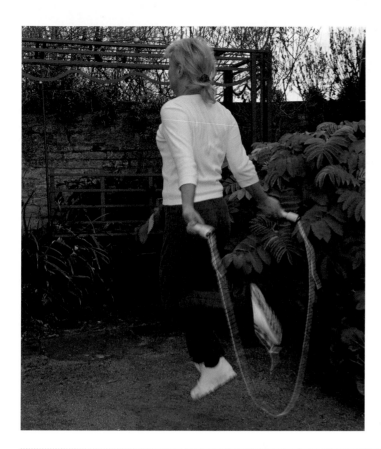

Skipping with a rope is a great way to burn calories on a flat surface in the garden. Gravel and grass work especially well. To optimize fitness benefit, stand with your back in neutral and your abdominal muscles pulled up and in. Your head should be facing straight ahead.

Back Extensions

When doing back extensions, your deep stabilizing muscles must work to support your lower back. If you have any back problems, you should consult a professional before attempting this.

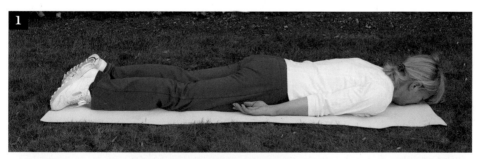

1 Lie on your front, with your arms by your sides. Inhale and draw in your lower abdominal muscles.

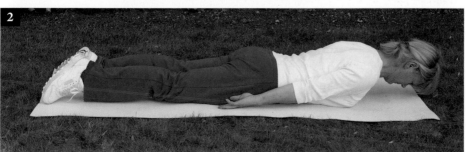

2 Exhale and gently lift your head and shoulders. Avoid arching your back. Hold for a few seconds, then gently lower yourself back down and repeat.

Outdoor Dynamic Workouts

Abdominal Curls

When it comes to abdominal exercise, it is absolutely crucial to get the technique right. Make every effort not to hold your breath, and do not push your belly out at any point (as this fails to support the back, and also defeats the purpose of sculpting and flattening your abdomen). Also, you should never lurch forwards; this is essentially 'cheating', as the momentum will be doing the work rather than your abdominals.

All of these abdominal exercises should be done slowly and with control—after all, the time spent working your abdominals, as well as the quality of the movement, is more important than the number of repetitions you do. This control should come from your deep muscle system, so if you have learned to engage your deep stabilizing muscles (as described in Chapter 1), you will get far more benefit from your abdominal workout.

If you have ever had abdominal surgery such as a caesarean section, suffer from back pain or incontinence, or have recently given birth, you should seek professional advice before abdominal exercise. Once you learn to engage your deep muscles you will feel the difference between deep and superficial abdominal work.

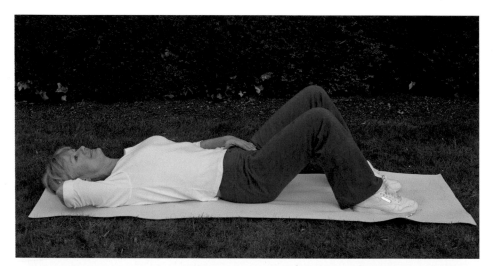

STARTING POSITION
Lie in the starting position: feet flat and knees bent, with one hand on your pelvis and the other behind your head.

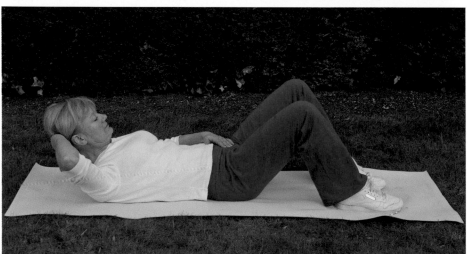

THE NORMAL CURL
Breathe in, and as you breathe out lift up your deep lower tummy muscles and curl forwards, taking care not to pull on the back of your neck. Curl up only as far as you can go with your back remaining in neutral. Hold and then lower.

THE OBLIQUE CURL
Use one hand to support the back of your head and the other hand to reach forward and touch the opposite knee. Your deep, lower abdominal muscles are lifted up. Your knees remain in alignment.

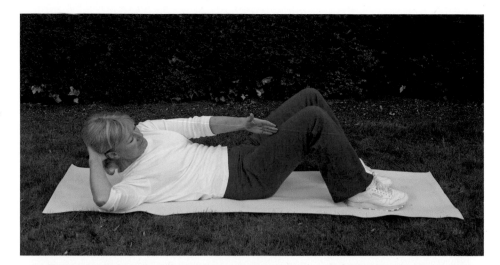

THE REVERSE CURL
Reverse curls should be done slowly and with control. Avoid this exercise if you have back problems or osteoporosis.

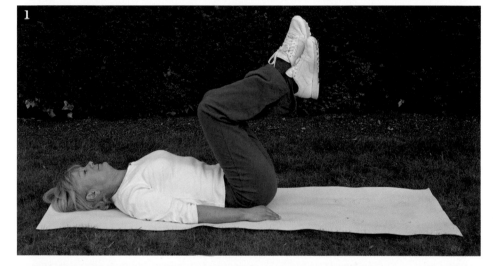

1 Begin in starting position, but with your hands resting down by your sides. Be careful not to push on them. Inhale and use your lower abdominals to lift your legs up, one at a time.

2 Exhale and lift up your lower abdominal muscles as you curl and lift your bottom off the ground, resisting the urge to curl up too high. Then, slowly lower your legs.

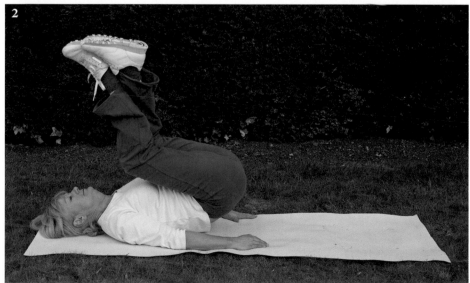

Balance and Strengthening

The following exercises involve bringing fitness equipment into the garden. They will help to tone your muscles, and will improve the sense of balance that is such an asset for gardeners.

USING FOAM ROLLERS

Bringing foam rollers, a small weighted ball, and a Pilates mat out into the garden will allow you to practise this powerful and deceptively difficult movement. This is Bunny's favourite exercise for developing core muscles, and if you spend long periods working at a desk you will find it especially satisfying (and even enjoyable) as you feel your core abdominal muscles at work.

The foam roller shown here is D-shaped, but you can also use circular foam rollers of various diameters which give a more challenging workout. If you have back or neck problems or are pregnant, you should skip this exercise. It is well worth seeking out a Pilates studio that uses this equipment so that they can supervise you initially.

Arm Lowering

Begin by lying on the D-shaped section of the foam roller. Gradually build up to 10 on each side, going only as far as you can with your torso still and centred.

• **Be careful not to brace the back of your neck while you initiate the movement.**
• **This movement should stem from your pelvic floor and lower abdominals. Do not tighten your abdominals at any point.**

1 Lie on your back with your head and bottom on the foam roller. Place your hands up in the air with your palms together; find neutral alignment of your spine. Inhale.

2 Exhale, pulling your pelvic floor and lower abdominals up and in while lowering one arm towards the ground. Then slowly return to the starting position.

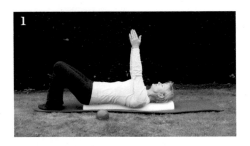

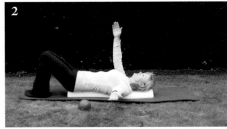

Using a Weighted Ball

Once you familiarize yourself with the basic movement, you can move on to incorporating the weighted ball. When you start, make sure that you feel stable on the foam roller before you commence the exercise. Your back should not be arching, and your abdominal muscles must not bulge outwards. Work up to 10.

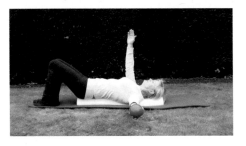

Repeat as above, but hold the weighted ball in your hands. Perform the movement slowly and with control. Avoid twisting your torso, and remember that your lower abdominals are being challenged.

Knee Drops

As you perform Knee Drops, your core muscles must work continuously in order for your pelvis to remain still as your knee drops to one side. Try closing your eyes; when you lose your vision, on which you rely to stay balanced, you challenge your core balance still further. Work up to 10.

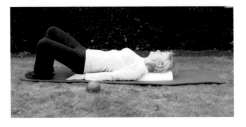

Inhale. Exhale and pull your pelvic floor and lower abdominal muscles up and in as one knee opens slowly to the side before returning to centre. Your pelvis stays still, strong, and stable.

SWISS BALL EXERCISES

Swiss Ball exercises are wonderful for challenging your balance and strengthening your deep stabilizing muscles. Though the balls are fun, they are also very challenging to use properly.

Because a Swiss Ball is inherently unstable, you will probably find yourself wobbling around, holding your breath, and bracing in order to maintain stability. When you first start using the Swiss Ball your challenge will be to avoid and overcome these 'cheating' mechanisms as they can lead to overusing the superficial, global muscles instead of the local, stabilizing muscles that you should be targeting. It is important to start slowly and progress carefully until your deep muscle system begins to respond to the inherent instability of the ball in an automatic, relaxed, and coordinated way.

By using the Swiss Ball with proper technique, your body will eventually learn to remain relaxed and balanced in its movements. In time this leads to more fluid and dynamic movement.

The exercises work out your entire body. The roundness of the ball means you can move your body forwards and backwards, and side to side, and in circular movements. This last manoeuvre takes a lot of concentration and should not be attempted until your muscle control is well developed. In the physiotherapy clinic, rotational exercises on the Swiss Ball are wonderful for twisting motions in the garden such as raking and compost digging. They also help to ease off stiffness after gardening.

Using the ball can be mental as well as physical work; it can be used as a tool to stretch, to breathe, to stabilize, and to relax. You may wish to run through the following sequence as one of your weekly outdoor workouts, but you can also substitute some ball exercises for certain elements on the workout 'menu' on page 45—for instance, do your curl-ups on the ball rather than on the ground.

Choosing Your Swiss Ball

These exercise balls were initially designed and manufactured by Aquilino Cosani in Italy in 1963. They were first put into clinical use by the Swiss paediatrician Dr. Elsbeth Kong along with Mary Quinton, a British-trained physiotherapist who specialized in the Bobath Technique for treating neurological conditions in hospitals for children. Since then, many physiotherapists have written books that explore the usage of Swiss Ball exercises for treating a range of conditions. They are now used outside of the medical setting for fitness purposes.

These balls come in many different forms; different manufacturers have different standards and as usual you tend to get what you pay for. Make sure the ball is sturdy enough to sustain your weight. It should be made of a plastic that will not burst, but instead deflate slowly if punctured—or, better still, it is worth seeking out one that is burst-resistant. It is crucial that your Swiss Ball be suitable for outdoor use. To protect it from damage, avoid exposing it to direct heat and sunlight.

The average Swiss Ball is usually just over 2 ft. (65 cm) tall. You should be able to sit on the ball with your hips and knees almost at a right angle, and your back in neutral.

SWISS BALL SAFETY

While using the Swiss Ball promotes health, it can also be dangerous. As with other exercises, you must stop immediately if you feel pain. It is a good idea to check with your doctor before working with the ball.

Working on a mobile surface means that the exercises are more challenging for your body, so it is very important to build up gradually through the movements and never to rush them. Balance and control require concentration and endurance. Initially, just sitting on the ball might be enough of a workout. If you are unfit or recovering from an injury you will need to take it very slowly. Some people might suffer from vestibular problems (symptoms include lightheadedness and trouble balancing), or motion sickness at first; this can sometimes be helped by starting with just one or two exercises before steadily building up to the full workout. Falling off the ball can cause serious injury so ensure your surface is not slippery. You might want to place an exercise mat on top of your garden surface, as it will stick to the ball very slightly and improve its traction.

Finally, try not to let children play with your Swiss Ball, especially unsupervised; although the balls may look like fun toys, it is all too easy for them to injure themselves by falling or slipping.

Balance and Strengthening

SIX SWISS BALL EXERCISES FOR GARDENERS

The six exercises shown here have been specifically chosen to benefit gardeners. They will help you to find neutral, move your upper body, strengthen your legs and abdominal muscles, lengthen your spine, and finally to maintain balance and strength while cultivating better alignment at the same time.

These exercises are deceptively tricky. Try to concentrate on keeping your back in its neutral position (neither distorted, nor slumped, nor arched) and your abdominal muscles engaged. This takes practice, but these movements are worth mastering and practising to build up core strength and coordination. Because the ball is unstable, you may feel inclined to overwork muscles in order to maintain balance. To counter this tendency, it helps to remind yourself that 'less is more'.

Pelvic Tilts

You should be able to feel the motion of your pelvis rolling back and forth as the ball moves beneath you. Because the ball's surface is soft you can relax your pelvic floor into the ball and then gradually lift it up. A series of 6 tilts will provide a good pelvic workout.

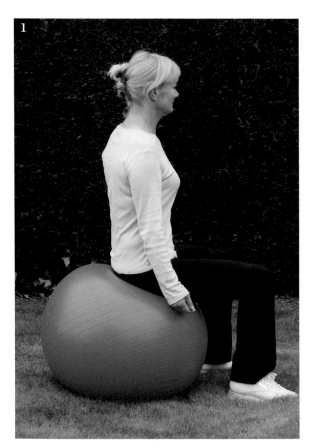

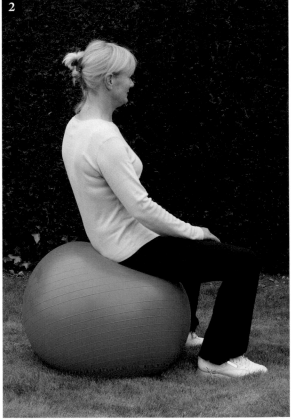

1 Begin by sitting on the ball, with feet flat on the floor, knees hip-width apart and spine in its neutral position. Your deep stabilizing muscles should be engaged. Your back should be upright in its neutral position.

2 Gently slump into the ball allowing your tailbone to sink into it. Then gradually straighten back up again, lifting your chest up but not sticking it out until you are back in neutral.

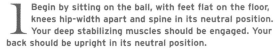

Twists

Twists are lovely for loosening up a stiff upper back. Only the top half of your back should move. Do 3 on each side.

Swiss Ball Squats

Swiss Ball squats will tone your bottom. To make this exercise more difficult, you can do it while standing on your toes. This calls for good balance and foot control (and is not recommended for those with weak ankles). Alternatively, repeating the same exercise with legs apart in a *plié* position will really work your inner thighs, buttocks, and hips. Do 6 slow repetitions.

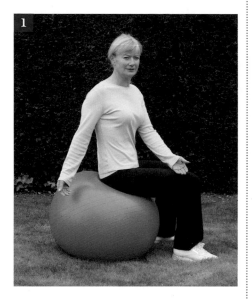

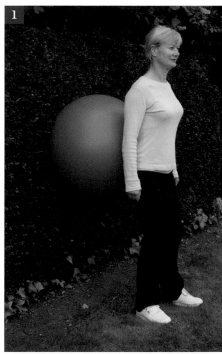

1 Begin by standing with the ball placed against a reasonably firm vertical surface in the garden. It should be positioned behind your lower back with your feet placed out in front of you, hip-width apart.

1 Begin in the starting position for Pelvic Twists. Place your arms by your sides. Breathe in, and as you breathe out lift your lower abdominals and pelvis up and in while lengthening your spine. At the same time, twist your upper body with your neck in one direction and place the opposite arm across the opposite knee.

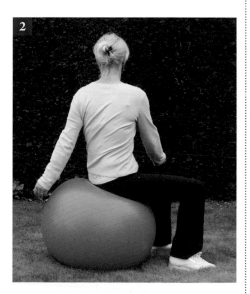

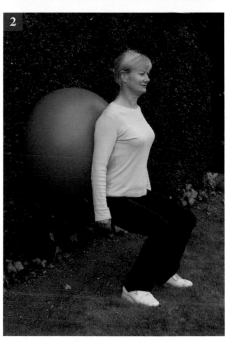

2 Breathe in and lower your knees so that your legs form an angle just over a right angle. Do not allow your knees to come together. Keep your feet aligned with your knees and do not let your knees lock. Finally, breathe out and straighten your legs.

2 Breathe in and slowly return to neutral. Then, twist to the other side. When you repeat, remember to alternate sides to get a balanced workout.

Balance and Strengthening

Swiss Ball Curl-ups

When performed on a Swiss Ball, Curl-ups work your lower abdominal muscles effectively. By resting your legs on the ball, your hip muscles are in a shorter position and this can help to stop them from overworking. This also allows you to focus on the deep muscles in your pelvic floor and lower abdominals.

It is actually quite difficult to focus on your lower abdominals and resist the temptation to overuse these muscles as the ball on which your legs are resting 'gives' a little bit during the curling up motion. Keep your legs relaxed. When you curl up, do not push your heels hard into the ball as this may cause your hamstrings to overwork and tighten.

As you curl up (and then back down again), imagine that your spine is lengthening. Your pelvis should not twist during the curl, and your back should remain in its neutral position as you lift up your pelvic floor and lower abdominals. Your stomach should not bulge out at any point. Aim for 10 repetitions.

1 Lying on your back, place the ball under your legs so that your calves rest on top of it. Place one hand behind your neck to support it and put your other hand on your pelvis to make sure it does not twist throughout the exercise.

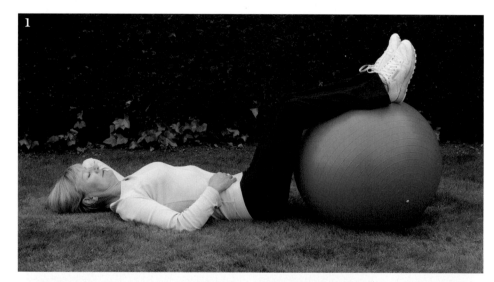

2 Breathe in and on the breath out pull your pelvic floor and lower abdominal muscles up and in, gently curling up.

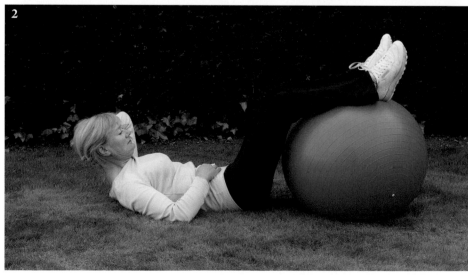

Side Stretch

This exercise will give you a lovely stretch at the side of your body. Your back should stay neutral. Maintain your balance and control as you change position. Carry out 5 stretches on each side.

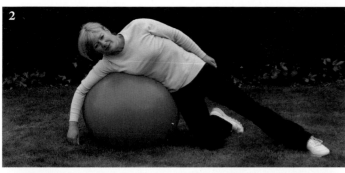

1 Lie over the ball on your side, with your right leg bent and your right arm following the curve of the ball. Your left leg should be extended to provide stability, and your left arm resting by your side.

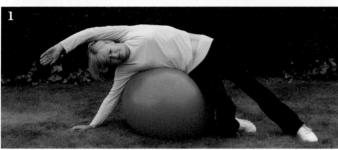

2 Inhale deeply and slowly, feeling your ribs expand. Exhale and let your left arm float up and over your head. Then, roll onto your stomach and repeat on the other side.

Swiss Ball Press-ups

Swiss Ball Press-ups will tone and strengthen your arms. This exercise is difficult, especially if you do not naturally have much upper body strength. Gradually build up to 10 repetitions if you can.

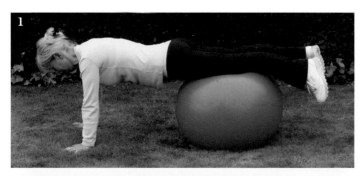

1 Lie on the ball, which should be placed just below your thighs. Your spine should be in neutral, your palms should be on the ground beneath your shoulders, and your neck should not be tightened or twisted as you face the ground.

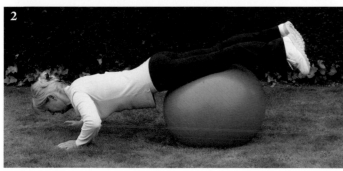

2 Breathe in to bend the arms and then breathe out and straighten them. (Do not hyperextend, or lock, your elbows). Focus on keeping your back in neutral as you lift up your pelvic floor and lower abdominals throughout the exercise. Work from your shoulder blades, and keep the back of your neck lengthened to avoid strain.

Trim Trail Exercises

Installing a miniature trim trail on virtually any garden surface—be it grassy or paved, completely flat or set on different levels (see Chapter 4)—will create a very personalized workout space.

One option is an exercise beam, which you can use for a variety of balancing and toning exercises. A stretching area, consisting of posts of different sizes set into the ground, is also useful. In the garden you can improvise, using sturdy steps, benches, trees, or even large rocks.

You can also use your trim trail as part of a circuit training routine by running around it before stretching on it. It need not be anything more complicated than a step-up log and a path.

Site it carefully, in a spot that you find pleasant and stimulating. A woodland clearing or shelterbelt (see Chapter 5) is a wonderful place for this kind of exercise equipment, and if you are lucky enough to have a spot in your garden that overlooks an inspiring view, this is a real bonus.

A bench is a great place for a leg lengthening stretch after a strenuous gardening session.

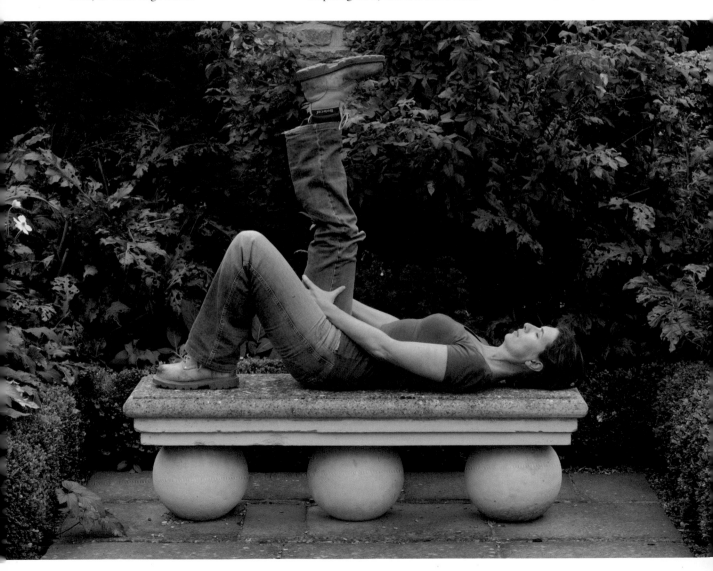

USING AN EXERCISE BEAM

Installing an exercise beam is a great way to turn a garden spot into a personalized outdoor gym. It is a versatile piece of equipment which can form the basis for a challenging outdoor workout. Ideally it should be no higher than 20 in. (0.5 m); anything higher is a safety risk when used as a balance beam—although it is possible to break an arm falling from even a very low beam, so do be careful. The width of the beam should be 4–5 in. (10.3–12.8 cm). Using this contraption, you can train both your upper and lower body and practise engaging your deep stabilizing muscles by completing the series of exercises below.

Balancing

Babies learn to balance automatically and intuitively. When they reach out to grab things, they fall over when they get it wrong but with practice and repetition they learn where their limits lie and slowly gain control.

Our bodies are naturally inclined towards improving balance, and balancing on a beam in the garden is a wonderful way to tune into the deep muscle system. When you feel you are losing your balance and wobbling a little, your arms go out to your sides and you use your deep stabilizing muscles to keep you upright and retain your balance.

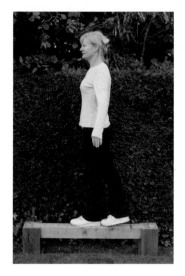

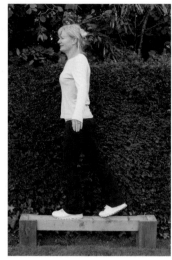

A good way of balancing is to walk along one foot in front of the other. You can walk along slowly, moving heel to toe so that each foot touches the one in front.

Once you have built up your balancing ability, take bigger, quicker steps across the beam. This challenges and sharpens your coordination.

Arabesques

Doing Arabesques on your exercise beam is another way to work your deep stabilizing muscles and improve your balance. This is a challenging exercise; start by holding the position for 10 seconds and gradually work your way up to a full minute.

You may find that you have better balance on one side of the body than the other. To cultivate good balance it is a good idea to practise walking across the beam with your left foot leading if you are right-handed, or vice versa.

Begin standing on one leg atop the beam, and bend the knee of your supporting leg very slightly. Lean forwards at your hip with both arms out to the side and bring your other leg straight out behind you. Hold your balance for a count of 60 and then lower your extended leg back onto the beam.

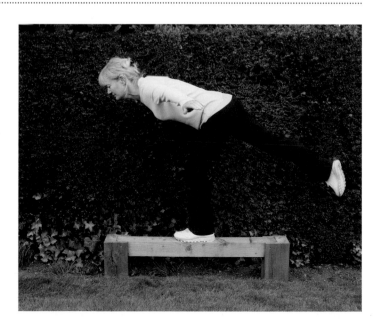

Trim Trail Exercises

The following exercises make use of an exercise bench, but you can also use a lower table or even a fallen log in the garden—just be sure that it is completely stable! Completing the entire sequence will give you a workout, improving your balance, coordination, and muscle tone. Begin with 8 repetitions of each exercise, building up to 10 and then 15 as your level of fitness improves.

Press-ups

Press-ups may feel difficult at first; if so, start by bending your knees and resting them on the ground so that your arms are only supporting half of your body weight. It is important to keep your body in alignment, with your hands directly underneath your shoulders.

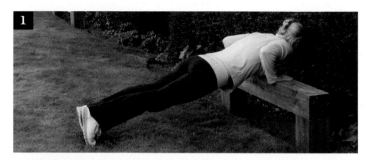

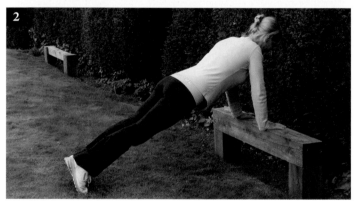

1 Begin with your body in a diagonal line against the bench, with elbows bent and legs straight but not locked. Your elbows should form a right angle.

2 Press up with your arms so that they are straight but not locked. Keep your back and neck straight and your stomach pulled in. Your body should stay in a nice, straight line even as you lower yourself back down and repeat.

Dips

Dips are a great way to define the backs of your arms. As you dip, take care not to let your shoulders fall forward as this will place too much much strain on your shoulder joints.

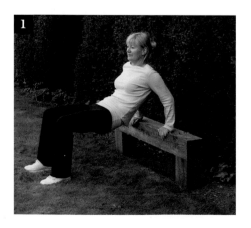

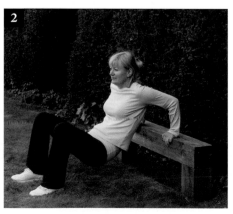

1 Start facing away from the bench with your feet on the ground, your knees bent at a right angle, your arms on the bench behind you and your bottom suspended.

2 Slowly bend your elbows, keeping the rest of your body still and straight as you lower it gradually. Keep your abdominal muscles continuously lifted. Then slowly straighten your arms as your body is raised.

Power Lunges

Power Lunges are particularly effective for toning your bottom. They also challenge your sense of balance.

1 Stand in front of your exercise beam with your back to it. Bend one knee back and place your foot on the beam while keeping the other on the ground. Your arms can be out at your sides for balance.

2 Bend your front knee and lean forward. Keep your back straight and your supporting knee facing forward—it should not wobble or twist. Pull in your lower abdominal muscles and use your gluteal muscles to help you return to starting position.

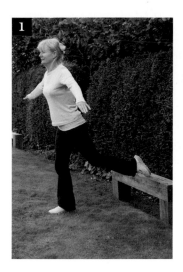 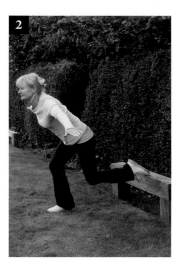

Bridging

Bridging builds up your balance and deep muscle control. As an advanced variation, try lifting one foot off the bench while your back is raised off the ground. You may want to perform Bridging on a Swiss Ball in addition to the beam to further challenge your control and balance.

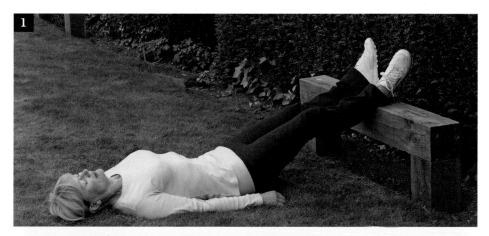

1 Begin lying on your back, with your feet on the bench and your spine in neutral. Hook your heels around the far edge of the beam. Inhale to prepare.

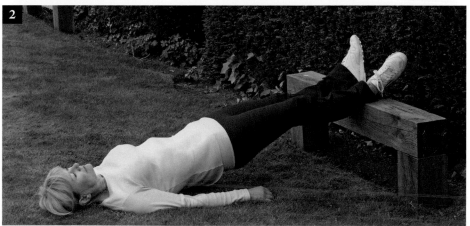

2 Exhaling, use your pelvic floor and lower stomach muscles to raise your back off the ground, being careful not to overarch your spine. Hold for a few seconds before lowering.

Trim Trail Exercises

USING YOUR STRETCHING POSTS

It makes sense to install a series of three stretching posts with different heights, as this will allow you to vary the level of difficulty of your stretching routine.

If you are of average height, your middle post should be around 1.5 ft. (45 cm)—but there is no hard and fast rule. As can be seen in the photographs in the following pages, different stretches may be suitable for posts of different heights. However, do be careful not to strain your muscles by trying to use the highest possible stretching post when you may not be flexible enough to get into this stretch.

The posts shown here measure approximately 6 × 6 in. (15 × 15 cm) in surface area. They extend around 1 ft. (30 cm.) into the ground and have some concrete at their base that serves to hold them in place.

From a design perspective, you can turn stretching posts into an asset by forming a series of posts into a see-through fence. Stretching posts fit in well towards the front of an informal border or an area of low planting. Avoid placing them in grass, as they tend to be a nightmare to mow around. If you are constructing them yourself, it is best to use hardwood timber or softwood that has been pressure-treated with preservative.

The following stretches may be done in lieu of the leg lengthening, hip loosening, and thigh stretches detailed in Chapter 1. Remember to stretch only after an active gardening or exercise session, when your muscles are warm and malleable; never stretch when your muscles are cold, before you have carried out any physical activity.

As with many of the stretches described earlier in the book, these stretches should each be held for 30 seconds to a minute. Generally you should carry out a series of 3 stretches on one side and then switch to the alternate side to perform 3 more.

You can use softwood stretching posts like these to double up as an informal fence.

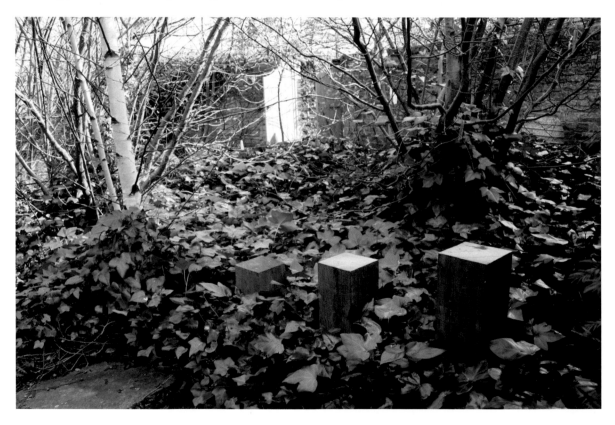

Hamstring Stretch

You will feel the Hamstring Stretch in the back of the thigh of your leg that rests on the post as you straighten it.

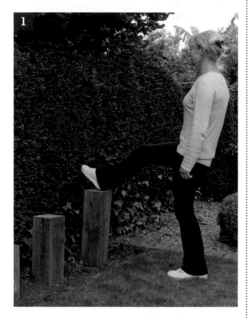

1 Begin standing up in front of the post with your back in neutral. Place the heel of one leg on the post, with your knee bent. Your supporting leg should be straight but not locked.

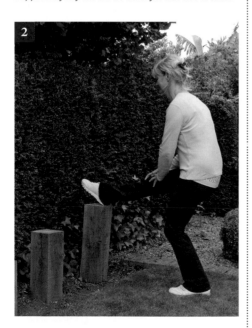

2 Lean downward into the stretch and slowly straighten your knee. Release by bending your knee, with your back remaining upright.

Hip Stretch

The Hip Stretch is felt around the hip of your supporting leg. Try to keep your back upright even as your body is leaning forward. Do not twist at the waist.

Begin standing in neutral in front of the bench. Then, place one foot on the edge of the post and lean gently forwards into your bent knee with your lower abdominals lifted and your pelvis facing forward. Release the stretch by returning to an upright position.

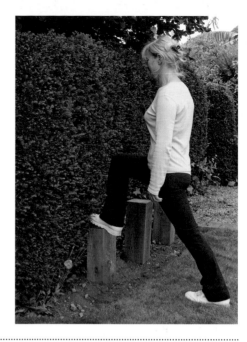

Quadriceps Stretch

This Quadriceps Stretch requires that you practise good balance. The thigh of the leg resting on the post will feel the stretch. Try to keep your back still throughout the stretch, resisting the temptation to arch it towards your back leg. It is harder than it looks!

Stand in neutral with your back to the post. Place one leg on the post behind you so that this back knee is bent at a right angle. Slowly bend the knee of your supporting leg as you lower yourself, keeping your pelvis straight and drawing your lower abdominals in as you engage your deep stabilizing muscles. Then slowly straighten your supporting knee.

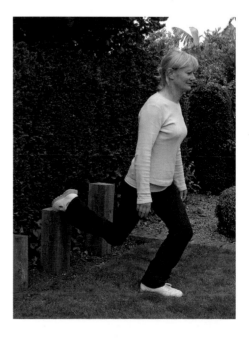

Winding Down

At the end of a gardening session, taking a few minutes to practise deep, relaxed breathing in a pleasant spot has a wonderfully soothing effect. In addition to helping your body to wind down after a bout of dynamic exertion, studies have shown that relaxed, meditative breathing can have a positive effect on mental health, helping to reduce anxiety and depression.

WHAT IS HEALTHY BREATHING?

Healthy breathing involves taking in air with minimal effort, in a way that makes efficient use of your respiratory muscles. These include the diaphragm, the intercostal muscles, and the accessory muscles of respiration.

Although breathing happens automatically, our rate and depth of breathing may be altered for various reasons such as smoking, chest conditions, stress, anxiety, and poor posture. If breathing is affected by such factors over long periods of time, we learn bad breathing habits. When we become stressed or anxious, we may develop tension in the neck and shoulders and our breathing can in turn become quicker and shallower. This is inefficient, as we tend to then use only the upper part of our lungs. Shallow breathing leads to an inefficient exchange of carbon dioxide and oxygen, which can leave us feeling exhausted. The same applies to poor posture; if we sit slumped at a desk all day, then our lungs can become slightly compressed. If we use the phone at the same time, then we have a tendency to gulp in air while talking which results in short, rapid breathing.

People with pathological and/or long-term bad breathing patterns must seek medical advice to pinpoint the underlying cause. Respiratory physiotherapists can train you to breathe properly. The advice provided here is simply a guide to help you to find a healthier breathing pattern.

BREATHING FOR RELAXATION

We tend to breathe too rapidly when we are stressed. A healthy rate of breathing is ten to fourteen breaths per minute, and as you relax, you will find that your rate of breathing lowers. After you have been relaxing and concentrating on your breathing for a few minutes, try counting the number of breaths you take each minute: ten breaths per minute is an ideal pace for relaxation. Rather than taking in big gulps of air, concentrate on the fresh air filling your abdomen and lower ribcage.

- **Shrug your shoulders before you begin; they should not be hunched up towards your neck. This helps to release tension in the muscles of respiration.**
- **Release your jaw so that there is no tension in your neck or face. Allow your brow to soften, too.**
- **Your lips should be together to encourage nose breathing, but they should not be clamped tightly shut.**
- **Breathe air in through your nose gently, allowing it to expand your stomach. Do not force it; it should feel effortless.**
- **You may want to place your hands on your ribcage as it fills with air and recedes.**

MIND AND BODY

When you are winding down, your exhalation should ideally be twice as long as the inhalation - but do not get caught up in counting the seconds. Instead, focus on the melting away of any stress or anxiety that may be lurking in your body or mind as you breathe out.

To concentrate on the out breath, practise breathing out from the back of your throat. This will make a slightly husky sound as you exhale.

Imagine a weeping willow tree with its branches swaying in the breeze. Try to make your breathing as rhythmic as possible to match the way this tree might flow back and forth in the wind.

RIGHT: Take some time to unwind in your favourite garden spot.

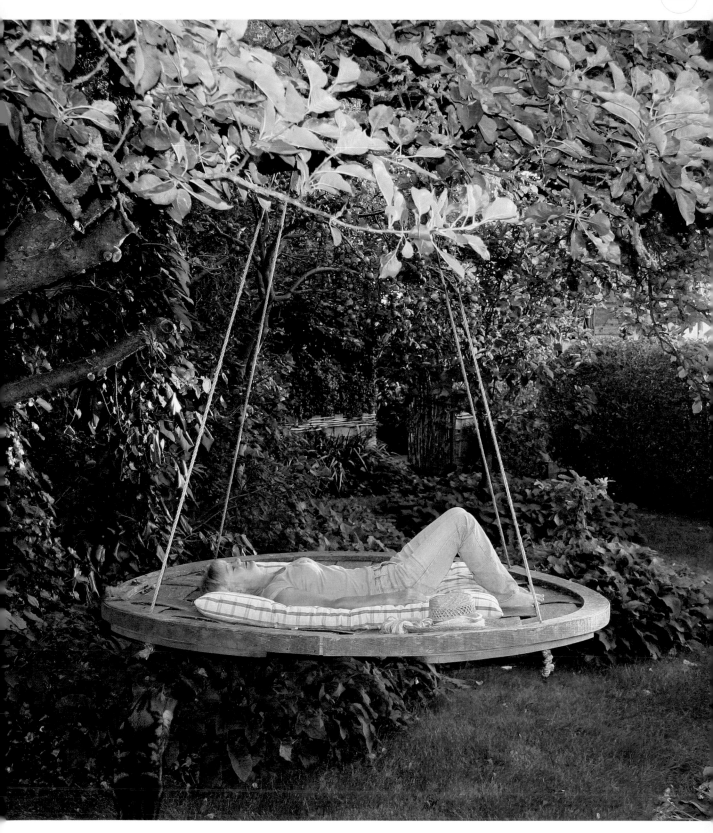

Winding Down

POSITIONING YOURSELF

A number of different positions are conducive to relaxed breathing in the garden. Choose whichever position makes you feel most relaxed.

Sitting and leaning over is a good position for winding down. (Alternatively, the odd tree trunk comes in handy for deep relaxed breathing: sit or kneel on the ground and lean forwards, draping your arms around the tree trunk.) Allowing your stomach to fall forward encourages deeper breathing as you draw air into your lungs; in this position, you are more inclined to relax your upper chest and accessory muscles of respiration.

You may find it most relaxing to breathe while lying on your back. Lying on top of a blanket will help you to relax into the surface beneath you, releasing any unwanted tension that may exist in your muscles. You can also recline on a lounger, opening up the front of your chest.

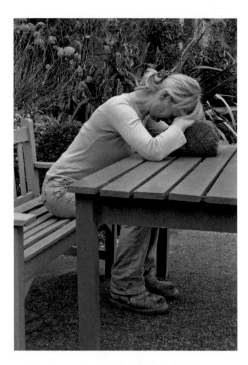

SITTING AND LEANING
Try sitting at a comfortable chair beside a table in the garden, leaning forward onto the table. It is a good idea to use a pillow for support.

LYING DOWN
This is the most relaxing deep breathing position of all. Imagine your body melting into the surface beneath you.

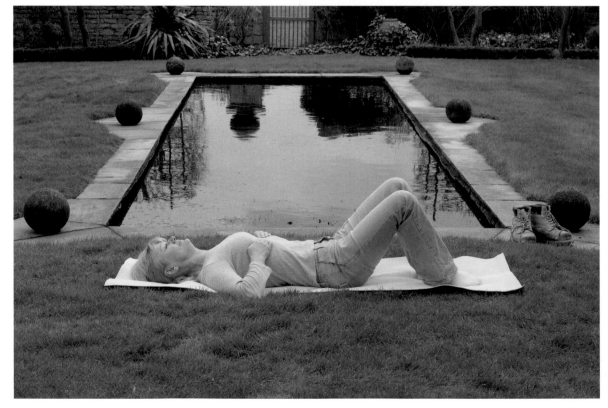

LOUNGING
Reclining on a lounger is a particularly attractive option after a demanding gardening session. This position allows the front of your chest to be open, the opposite of slumped.

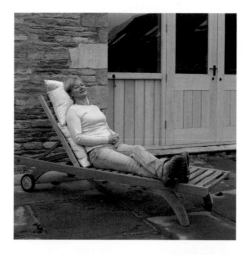

A major benefit of unwinding outside is that the sensory stimuli in the garden can bring about a sense of wellbeing. Of course, scent is important and if you can situate yourself next to some fragrant flowers or herbs this will be an added bonus. In particular the scent of lavender is thought to have a relaxing, and even sedative, effect. (See Chapters 5 and 6 for details on growing lavender for ornamental value and aromatherapeutic benefits, respectively.)

Any sound that is slow and fluid can help you to focus on your breathing. The sound of water, wind, or a birdsong can help you to visualize the air moving in and out of your lungs as you settle into a very relaxed rhythm.

Better breathing technique can take a while to develop and it should never be rushed. The key is to allow yourself a few minutes to relax whenever you can, and to practise slow and relaxed breathing as often as possible. As with many of the exercises in this chapter, is is very possible to train yourself to develop better breathing habits through conscientious practice where you tune into what your body is telling you and treat yourself with good care.

If good breathing technique is practised regularly you will learn to breathe more efficiently throughout the rest of the day. It will also make you feel energized yet peaceful as you take the time to appreciate the garden around you.

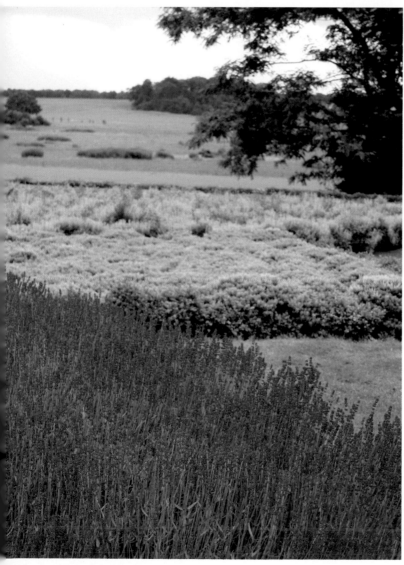

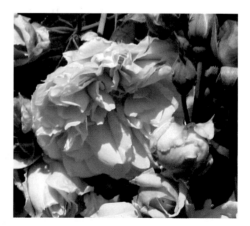

LEFT: If you can do your deep breathing next to a generous sweep of fragrant lavender, it may help you to wind down.

ABOVE: A sweet-smelling rose will enhance your relaxing experience.

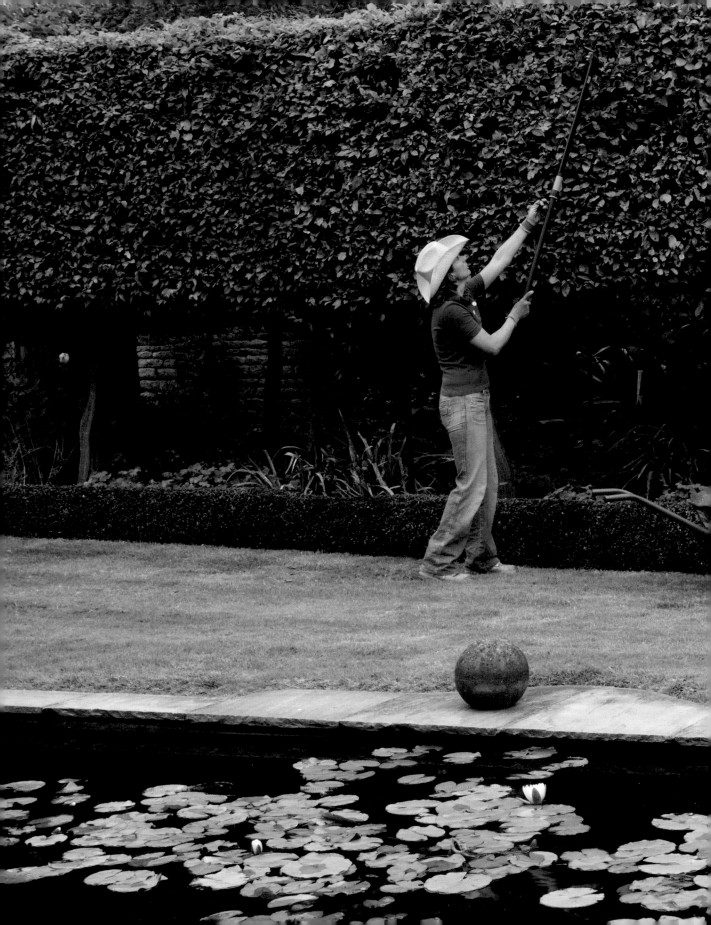

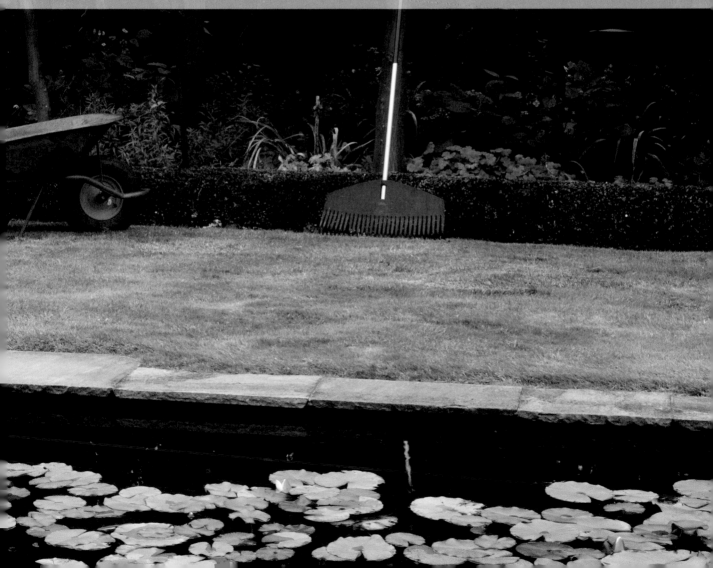

CHAPTER 3
SAFER GARDENING
tools and techniques

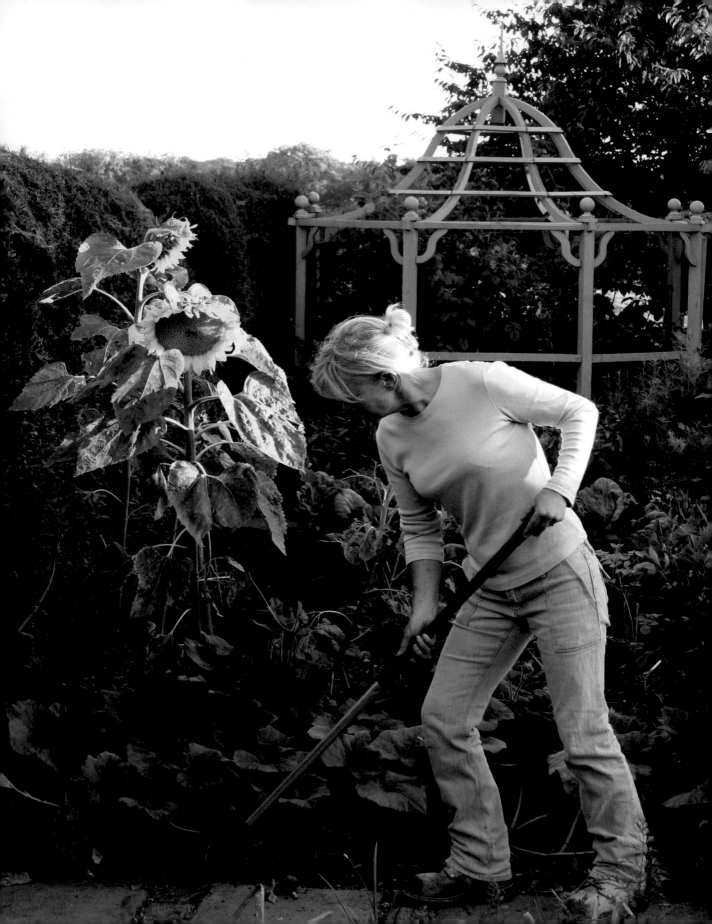

WHILE STRENGTHENING, stretching, and aerobic exercise help to build up the fitness and stamina necessary for gardening, the choices we make can exert a similarly powerful impact on how gardening makes us feel. Often we are creatures of habit when it comes to choosing garden tools, honing in on one or two favourites and then using them for the bulk of our gardening work. The postures we adopt, too, tend to become habitual so that in time the repetitive stooping, bending, and reaching we undertake can make us feel sore and prone to injury.

We should resist becoming too stuck in our ways. We all have certain gardening actions that irk us, whether they involve raking large areas, hunching over to pull out weeds, or reaching up to prune branches far overhead—and in most cases, there will be room for improving these actions through the use of better tools or technique. New, lightweight, and ergonomic gardening tools are coming onto the market constantly, and it is worth experimenting with new tools that can make gardening easier and more efficient, helping us to get the job done while lessening the risk of damaging our bodies in the process.

Understanding how your body responds to gardening's various movements will influence the choices you make. If you notice your lower back stiffening, your neck becoming sore, or your knee joints complaining, it is important to take a good look at how you tend to treat your 'problem areas' so that you can learn to care for yourself in a more conscientious way. By improving how you treat the parts of your body that are vulnerable to strain, you can greatly improve your experience in the garden so that in time you will feel invigorated and healthy, rather than worn out and sore, after a session spent tending to your outdoor space.

This Dutch hoe makes weeding easier. It has a long and lightweight handle and a stainless steel head that will not rust. The head is bevel-edged and sharpened to slice through weeds efficiently.

Cornerstones of Safe Gardening

Regardless of which tools you use, the following guidelines will help you to protect your body from injury in the garden.

1. PACE YOURSELF

Gardening injuries increase dramatically in the spring, after people have been taking a break from gardening during the colder months. This is no coincidence; diving into an intensive gardening session too suddenly is a primary cause of injury in the garden. Gardeners unaccustomed to activity during the winter months tend to launch into gardening in the springtime, overexerting themselves and lifting excessively heavy loads without taking steps to prepare their bodies for it by sufficiently warming up, doing their pre-gardening strengthening exercises, and stretching afterwards. If you are overly ambitious about how much exertion your body can handle, your muscles will often 'complain' the next day.

Try to carry out shorter gardening sessions on a fairly regular basis, tackling your gardening tasks steadily over time instead of frantically trying to fit everything in on one free afternoon. Remember that gardening is physically strenuous work, and to do it for long periods requires stamina. It is best to pace yourself, rather like a long-distance runner would.

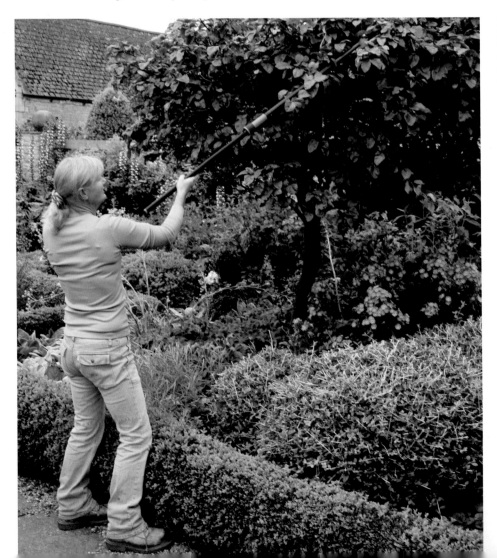

Long-reach, lightweight, and very effective, this telescopic universal cutter makes pruning far less strenuous.

2. BE AMBIDEXTROUS

Tasks like turning compost and raking leaves tend to involve favouring one side of the body, so that some muscles are built up while others become weak. Carrying out the body-balancing exercises described in Chapter 1 lays the groundwork for gardening in a more centred manner, but it also helps to be 'ambidextrous' as you complete your more lopsided gardening tasks. Raking with your non-dominant hand is definitely challenging, but with practice it is possible to adapt and it becomes easier. Whenever possible, try to change sides frequently, and if you are right-handed, use your left hand to pick things like weeds or low-lying fruit off the ground. Once you get past the initial strangeness of this temporary ambidexterity, it is a clever way of maximizing fitness benefits while protecting yourself from strain and injury.

Bodies love symmetry and balanced, coordinated movement. It takes time for the brain to relearn movement; in this sense, it is rather like learning another language. If you make a conscious effort to use the muscles on both sides of your body, then it follows that you will learn to become more centred and more aware of your body and its movement. The phrase 'if you don't use it, you lose it' may be a cliché, but it is altogether apt when it comes to the strength of your muscle system.

3. STAY HYDRATED

Bodies work better when they are well hydrated. Drinking enough fluid will protect you from the effects of dehydration, and it is also likely to give you more stamina and energy in the garden. Because dehydration can lead to increased muscle stiffness after a period of exercise, taking steps to stay hydrated is a vital way to safeguard yourself against feeling the worse for wear after a more intensive gardening session.

As soon as you start to feel thirsty, this means that your body is already dehydrated and needs a glass of water as soon as possible. If you are planning to work hard or for long periods of time, remember to bring a bottle of water or a pitcher of lemonade out into the garden with you. (Water is the best option for health-conscious gardeners, but natural fruit drinks without refined sugar are good alternatives.)

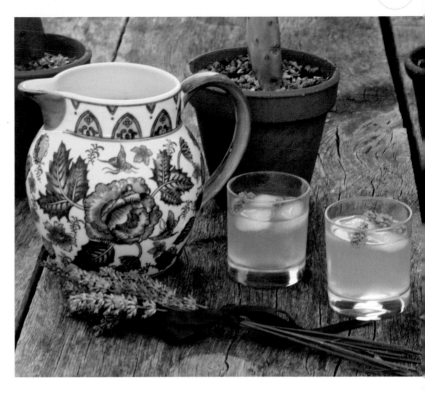

4. KNOW WHEN TO STOP

Many gardeners become so absorbed in the task at hand that they tend to ignore early warning signs of their joints or muscles becoming stressed. A growing sense of pain in your lower back or a stiffening neck is usually a sign that you need to take a break. If you keep going, you risk causing further damage and you may wake up the next morning feeling sore.

Bodies do not like sustained postures, especially when repetitive movement is involved. Treat yourself well by taking regular breaks (for instance, stroll around the garden with your back in neutral for a few minutes every quarter of an hour) and vary your activities as much as possible.

Think in terms of contrasting movements: a healthy body moves in all different directions, so if you have been bending of squatting for a while, you should move on to upright movements like standing or walking. Similarly, if you have been standing while potting for a while, your next movement might involve squatting or kneeling. Choosing ergonomic tools that encourage you to adopt healthier gardening postures can help you to avoid discomfort in the first place.

Iced lavender lemonade will keep you hydrated on hot days. (For the recipe, see Chapter 6.)

Knee Care

Gardeners commonly experience pain in their knees. Often it comes about after prolonged sessions spent kneeling or resting on all fours, during tasks such as weeding or picking low-lying fruit. The pain comes from sustained compression of the knee joints, which may inflame an underlying condition such as arthritis, or simply bring about new pain. (A less detrimental but nonetheless rather unnerving sensation of 'pins and needles' may also result when you rest on the backs of your shins as you kneel, cutting off blood supply to your lower legs.)

Generally speaking, knee pain in younger people tends to be caused by overuse, whereas in older people the pain is typically spurred by underuse. In both age groups, poor biomechanics can also play a role. People with osteoarthritis of the knee need to take special care not to put too much pressure on their knees while exercising. For instance, deep squats should be avoided.

The muscles at the fronts and backs of your thighs (the quadriceps and hamstrings, respectively) should work together to support your knee joints. Regular activity is key to achieving this. Because these muscles will tire quickly initally, it is best to start exercising slowly and build up gradually.

To avoid discomfort in your knees, avoid staying in a kneeling position for more than fifteen minutes at a time. It helps to take regular breaks and walk around your garden to help lubricate your knee joints. Indulging in a variety of contrasting types of movement is vital. For instance, if your time outdoors consists of a short bout of jogging, weeding on all fours, and then a series of lunges this variety of movement will benefit your body.

If you find yourself pushing on your thighs with your hands when you are moving out of a bending position, this might be happening because your thigh muscles are a bit weak. Alternatively, your thighs may be overworking in order to protect your back. If you have this tendency, you may gain a great deal of benefit from doing squats with good technique, as described in Chapter 2.

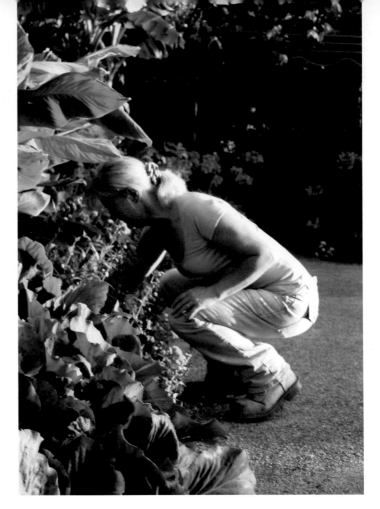

Ballet dancers are trained to turn their knees (and feet) outward, but the rest of us are prone to taking on postures that encourage our knees to roll inward. If we can concentrate a little on our knee alignment, then the stress that is placed on the knee joint and kneecap is often lessened. Try to avoid twisting your knee, and aim to keep your knees aligned by making sure that your kneecaps are directly above your second toes.

If you already have knee problems or find kneeling strenuous, it is a good idea to protect your knees with a support, or through wearing padded kneelers. Some gardeners may find traditional kneepads awkward to wear, as they often move and slip. However, it is possible to buy trousers that have built-in slots into which pads can be inserted, and you may find these to be more comfortable and effective than regular kneepads. Quite a few manufacturers make them for general workwear, and a Swedish firm called Snickers makes well-cut, hard-

When you squat to weed, keep your back in neutral and try to align your kneecaps over your second toes.

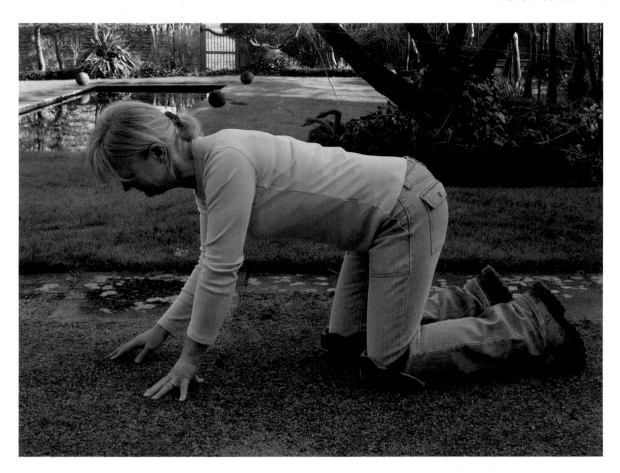

wearing yet stylish trousers and overalls
which can accommodate these
pads. Conveniently, they also have lots
of pockets and pouches in which you can
put knives, hand pruners (secateurs), seed
packets, and all the other essential bits
that you accumulate during your average
gardening session.

Feet and knees are closely related.
A supportive shoe or boot can help to
maintain the neutral position of your feet
which in turn will help to keep your knees
in alignment. When your feet twist or roll
inwards, this throws your knees out of
alignment and causes them to twist inwards
which places unnecessary force on your
knee joints and kneecaps which can lead to
discomfort and pain.

ABOVE: **Padded kneelers
take strain away from
your knees during
tasks like weeding in
gravel.**

RIGHT: **Squatting
while you sow seeds
is a great way of
maintaining hip
flexibility.**

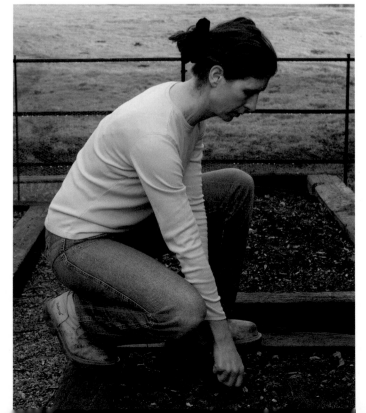

Shoulder and Neck Care

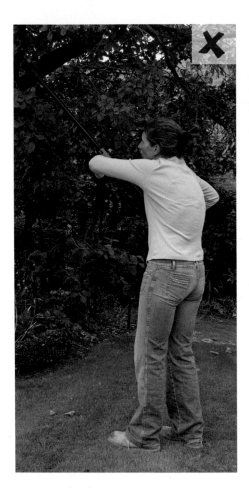

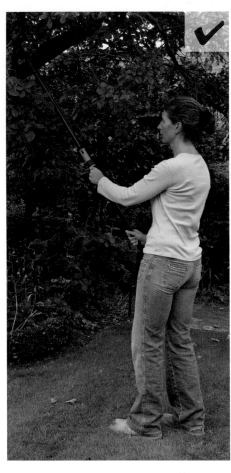

FAR LEFT: **Resist any temptation to hunch your shoulders and tense your neck.**

LEFT: **To avoid strain, keep your back in neutral and your neck and shoulders relaxed.**

For many gardeners, discomfort in the shoulders or neck is typically caused (and subsequently worsened) by overhead activities such as hedge trimming, watering hanging baskets, or pruning high trees. Your neck becomes particularly vulnerable to strain when you tilt it up to see what you are doing and then keep your neck in this position, as this position can result in compression of the neck joints. Similar strains can occur when you look up at stars or fireworks, or at the movie theatre or cinema when you are sitting too close to the screen. It is all too easy for gardeners to become so absorbed in a task that they forget to take breaks.

A great deal of tension and stress tend to be stored in the head, neck, and shoulders, and it is not always easy to let it go. Taking some time to walk around the garden as you shrug your shoulders up and down can really help to release this tension.

NECK CARE

The neutral position for the neck is where the head is balanced on top of the vertebral pillar, with the neck neither too far forward (with the chin sticking out) nor too far back. Visualize your head being like a football balanced on top of a pillar (the pillar being your backbone, or vertebral column).

When neck discomfort manifests itself, this is often related to an imbalance in the rest of the body, rather than just the head and neck. The foundations of good head and neck posture really start in the feet, in the base of the vertebral column, and in the pelvis. The way you hold your head and neck is related to alignment in your entire body, and problems tend to arise when the rest of the body is held in a position that is not entirely balanced.

Sometimes correcting head and neck alignment is not straightforward as the cause could be lower down. Whether or not you are predisposed to postural alignment will be due to a number of different factors including height, body type, genes, and your muscle tone.

Many methods exist which can help you to retrain your body so that you develop improved posture. The Alexander Technique has traditionally been used, and is still used today, to help correct postural alignment in musicians, and for the rest of us it is an excellent adjunct to the Pilates techniques described in Chapter 1. Certain types of yoga can also be very beneficial, as good alignment and correct breathing techniques are often integral parts of yoga classes. Those of us who have been instructed on good posture in school (that is, repetitively told not to slouch or stoop) have a distinct advantage. Of course, the body-balancing movements described in Chapter 1 will help you to realign the position of your head, neck, and shoulders; the Dart and the Diamond Press are particularly effective.

When you need to do overhead work in the garden, you can take steps to counteract neck and shoulder strain by adopting the following posture: stand in neutral with your back straight, your head balanced naturally on top of your neck and shoulders (rather than twisted), and your neck relaxed. Most importantly, your shoulders should be relaxed, rather than hunched up. It makes sense to use a small stepladder so that you are level with, or at least closer to, the tree you are cutting or the hanging basket that you are watering—just be sure it is stable and you do not fall off.

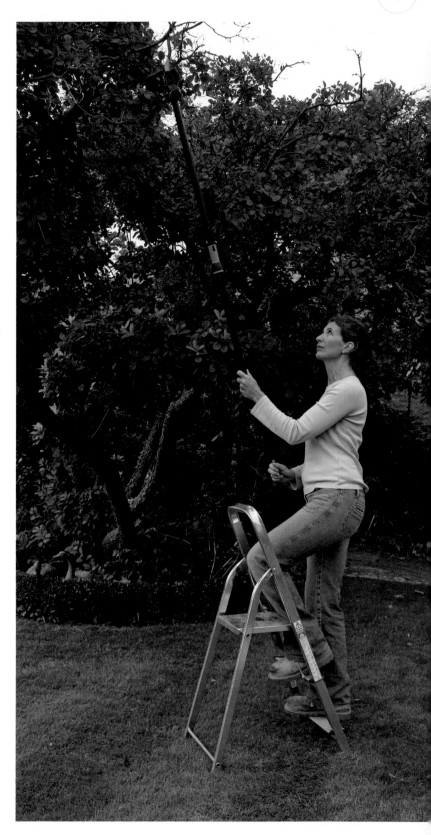

Using a small stepladder coupled with long-handled loppers reduces the need to tilt your neck backwards while pruning.

Shoulder and Neck Care

SHOULDER CARE

The way we experience shoulder movement is very closely tied to how our backs are aligned and how we hold ourselves in general. When we stand up straight there is a tendency to initiate the shoulder's movement from the shoulder blade, which is located at the back of the shoulder and has a close relationship with the spine.

Often gardeners feel strain in their shoulders when they carry out repetitive actions; raking, for instance, is a very common culprit. Try to take a break from this type of movement every ten minutes or so, and stop when you feel even a hint of discomfort in your shoulders. Make sure you are not hunching your shoulders or stooping over, and try to switch sides frequently. Do not carry out demanding repetitive activities like prolonged raking sessions without properly warming up.

To get a sense of the range of movement in your shoulders, try to take your arm forwards and up your head to almost 180°. Ideally, this should be easy and painless, but sometimes—normally due to rounded shoulders and poor posture—your shoulder joint movement becomes restricted so that it hurts to do this. If you start an activity and overuse some of the muscles that rotate the shoulder (the rotator cuff) then you may also find yourself unable to lift your arm out to the side without pain.

Many of the Pilates body-balancing exercises and post-gardening stretches detailed in Chapter 1 will benefit your shoulders, and on a daily basis it makes sense to move the shoulder joint through its full available range in order to stop it from stiffening up. This could be as simple as having a yawn and reaching up towards the sky, taking care not to overarch your back in the process.

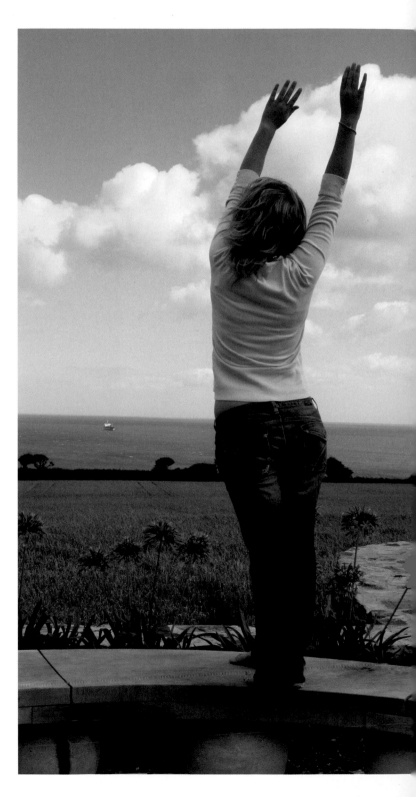

Reaching for the sky is a lovely stretch for the shoulders. Combining this with deep breathing and a wonderful view makes the experience even better.

Back Care

Back pain is such a common complaint among gardeners, and this is not surprising because common gardening actions like twisting, bending, and lifting in a way that strains the back can all engender discomfort and injury. Back pain can also come about when gardeners fail to pace themselves properly and attempt to do a job all in one go, when their bodies may not be prepared for it. Back pain can be particularly vexing as it can affect mobility.

Your spine is a long, S-shaped curve that runs all the way between your head and your tailbone. The base of the curve is the lower back (lumbar spine), which consists of five vertebrae. Above the lumbar spine is the thoracic spine, consisting of twelve vertebrae, and towards the top of the spine is the neck, or cervical spine, which encompasses seven more vertebrae.

These twenty-four vertebrae in the spine are all capable of movement. The vertebral column, or backbone, is supported by ligaments and a complex system of muscles. The deep layer of muscles tends to be responsible for holding your postural alignment, while the more superficial muscles relate to movement.

To help prevent back pain and relieve minor injury, it helps to focus on developing inner strength by targeting these deep muscles that are linked to posture. Doing the Pilates body-balancing exercises described in Chapter 1 will help you to strengthen these muscles, and the Swiss Ball exercises in Chapter 2 can help you move better. In addition to building inner strength by developing your deep postural muscles, honing your flexibility is also an essential element of back care. To this end, the post-gardening stretches described in the latter part of Chapter 1 will be beneficial.

If your pain is acute, this type of exercise should not be your first form of treatment—but it can certainly help to relieve chronic conditions.

Flexibility and strength are vital weapons against back pain and the only way to achieve them is to exercise regularly and develop your core muscles. To this end, any movement helps; try doing an aerobic regime outside, walking up and down steps, or jogging (as long as you pace yourself).

Finding neutral alignment of the spine, and then training your body to adopt the neutral position as you sit, walk, bend, and reach in the garden (as well as outside of it) can go a long way towards helping to prevent and help long-term back pain. Whenever you bend over in the garden, aim to keep your back as straight as possible while bending your knees, rather than leaning over from the waist, as this will help to take the load off of your spine.

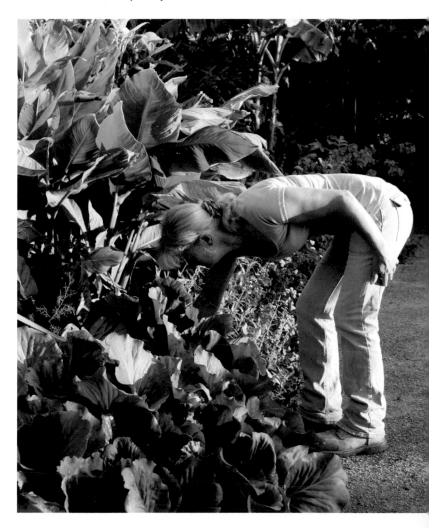

Bending from the waist is highly common among gardeners, but should be avoided when possible, as it can place additional stress on the spine. Avoid staying in this position for too long!

Stocking Your Toolshed

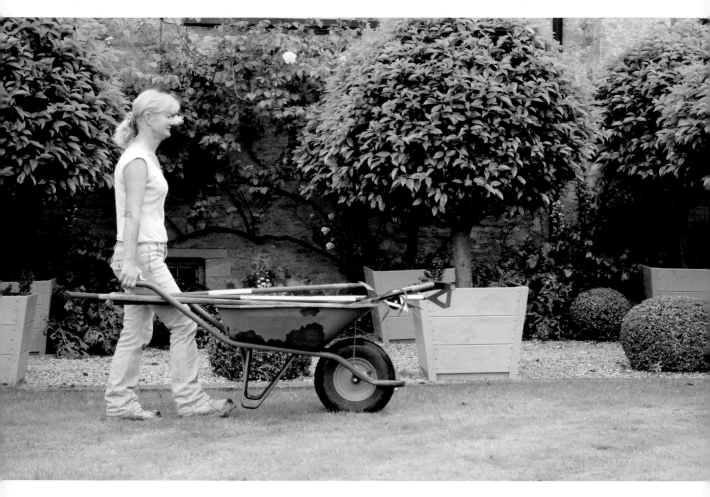

While some gardeners use a spade for lifting plants, others swear that a fork is better. We often hold very strong, or even stubborn, preferences about which tools are best for us. While it may be tempting to stick with a few tried and tested tools, it can be highly rewarding to try new things.

When seeking out tools, it is of course preferable to buy garden tools in person rather than over the internet as this lets you handle them to determine whether they fit well before you purchase. It is always good to try out a few different sizes and models, paying careful attention to whether the height, weight, and the length of their handles feel right, and whether they are too heavy to manoeuvre comfortably.

As a general rule, garden tools should be at a height that prevents you from having to take on uncomfortable positions like reaching too high for long periods or bending over awkwardly. For instance, your edger should come up to waist height so that you can work with your spine in neutral, and your wheelbarrow's handles should be large and high enough that you do not have to bend over too much, but can push loads through the garden while remaining upright.

Many manual tools such as strimmers (weed-whackers), trowels, hoes, rakes, spades, forks, and loppers are now available in long-handled versions. It is worth seeking these out as much as possible as they are

The handles of your wheelbarrow should have a length, width, and weight that lets you hold them without stooping or struggling.

often kinder to your spine in that they reduce the amount of bending, stooping, and reaching you need to do. They also help to relieve your neck and shoulders from this particularly strenuous position. Alternatively, add-on handles can be fitted onto the tools that you already have.

BASIC MANUAL TOOLS

The following are useful workhorses that deserve a place in the shed of any serious gardener.

Spades

Spades traditionally come in three sizes: a digging spade (large, usually with a broad blade); a ladies' spade (slightly smaller, and relatively lightweight); and a border spade (smaller and narrower). In addition, a new generation of longer, lighter spades which encourage you to adopt a more upright position are now on the market. Some also have an inward angle of 40° or so between the head and the shaft, which helps to maintain good posture.

The handle of the spade should reach up to your waist when you are standing up straight, to encourage your back to stay in its neutral position. If the spade is shorter, you will tend to stoop and hunch up more. The Wilkinson Power Border Spade (pictured on page 83) includes this feature. Despite having the word 'power' in its name, this spade is not motorized; it is a hand tool that has been ergonomically designed in order to make digging easier. It has a boron steel head so it is strong but soil does not stick to it, and includes a longer shaft.

Stainless Steel or Ordinary Steel Blade?

Whether you opt for a stainless steel blade or not will depend on how frequently you use your spade. If your spade will be spending long periods hanging on your potting shed walls, the stainless steel variety will stay smooth and so will slip through the soil with greater ease. An ordinary steel blade, on the other hand, is prone to forming a thin layer of rust on the surface if it is left unused for any length of time, and this rustiness tends to become clogged up with soil during use.

However, ordinary steel is stronger than the stainless variety, so if you are doing a lot of hard work ordinary steel is better. Many a stainless steel blade with a so-called 'lifetime guarantee' has been known to snap under the pressure of a heavy gardening boot!

Some spades have shoulders or small treads at the top of the blades. These are useful for cushioning your foot when you are doing a great deal of heavy digging. If your spade does not have this feature, ensure that your boots have strong, insulated soles that will protect and cushion your feet.

Whichever sort of spade you choose, keep its blade well sharpened. This will enable it to slice through turf and roots with far greater ease, saving you frustration.

Using an edger that comes up to waist height helps to maintain an upright posture. This lightweight half-moon edger has a stainless steel head with a sharpened bevel edge, and it slices through the turf with ease.

Stocking Your Toolshed

Fork

A fork is most useful when it comes to cultivating stony or heavy soil; compared to the blade of a spade, a fork's tines are far easier to push into the ground. Another advantage is that the fork will kill fewer worms in your soil. (Unfortunately, the notion that a worm split in two will automatically become two living worms is largely mythical; usually, only the end nearer to the head will stay alive, although some species are able to regenerate better than others.) Yet even though a fork breaks up soil more easily than a spade does, a spade is better for lifting up a small root ball as it will cause less damage.

It is worthwhile to buy two differently sized models. For intricate areas, a small, compact, and a light fork will serve you well, whereas larger areas with a cruder finish are best tackled with a bigger, beefier fork that you can really put your back into (as opposed to putting your back out, which is a real danger when you try to use an uncomfortably small fork for more heavy-duty tasks).

Pronged Cultivator

A pronged cultivator is useful for locally and lightly cultivating the surface layer of your soil before sowing seeds or planting in the vegetable garden. It is particularly

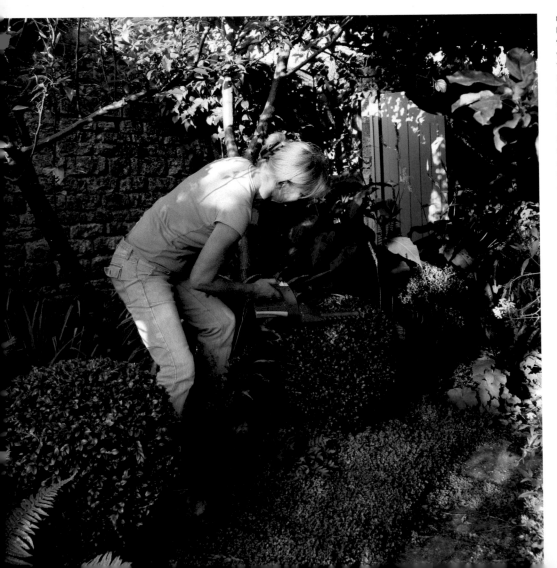

LEFT: These cordless, lightweight clippers take stress off of your wrists and hands. They need recharging intermittently, which stops you from doing one job for long periods of time.

RIGHT (FROM LEFT): An extra-wide rake (for collecting leaves and debris in large areas), a fork, a Dutch hoe, and a spade.

handy if you prefer the no-dig technique and want to let the worms do the work for you (for more information, see Chapter 4). Cultivators usually have between three and seven tines which are bent to form sharply pointed hooks. These are pulled through the soil in short, sharp movements as with the draw hoe, and it makes for quick and easily cultivating that does not unduly disturb the lower layers. That can be left to the plant roots, worms, and micro-organisms.

Wheelbarrow

In most gardens, wheelbarrows are indispensable. If you use one frequently, make sure it is efficient, allowing you to move quickly; if it is slow and difficult to push, it is probably time to buy a new one.

If you are bored with getting the pneumatic tyre mended because of thorny problems, you can get it fitted with a six-ply trailer tyre instead. This will stand up to years of rigorous wear and is not expensive.

Always try the wheelbarrow for size before you buy it, making sure that the handles are long enough that you don't hit your shins on the back of the barrow as you walk. The tray should be large enough for good-sized loads, too. Make sure it is narrow enough to fit through the narrow entranceways or paths in your garden.

If you have back problems, you may prefer to use a two-wheeled barrow. These are usually easier to manoeuvre and push than single-wheeled barrows, and they also seem to make the load feel lighter. However the two-wheeled barrows do not work as well on narrow paths.

Pruners (Secateurs)

Most gardeners live with a pair of pruners (secateurs) in their pocket. There are actually two types of pruners: those with bypass blades give a precise, clean cut and are ideal for new, green growth, while anvil pruners are efficient for cutting dry, hard, old growth. Some pruners come with finger loops that provide finger protection and are good for jobs that require a really secure grip. To ensure you do not inflict too much wear and tear on your pruners, try to avoid using them for large sections. It is a good idea to purchase a good pair of large, beefy loppers to tackle bigger sections of branch.

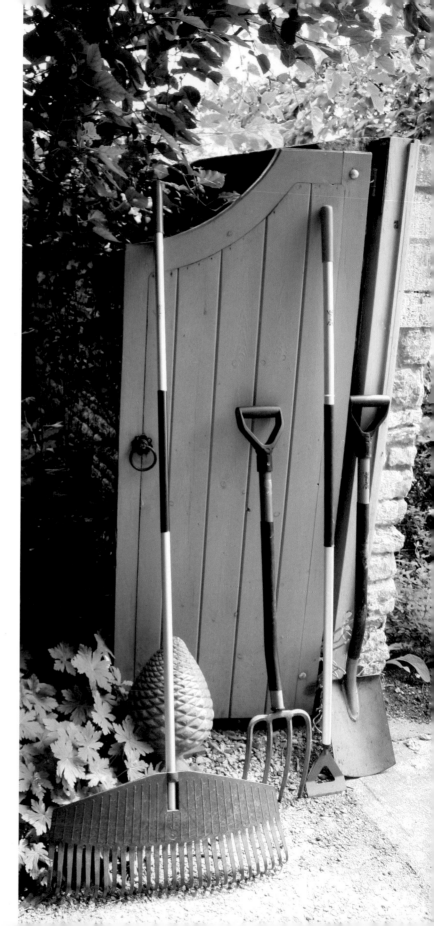

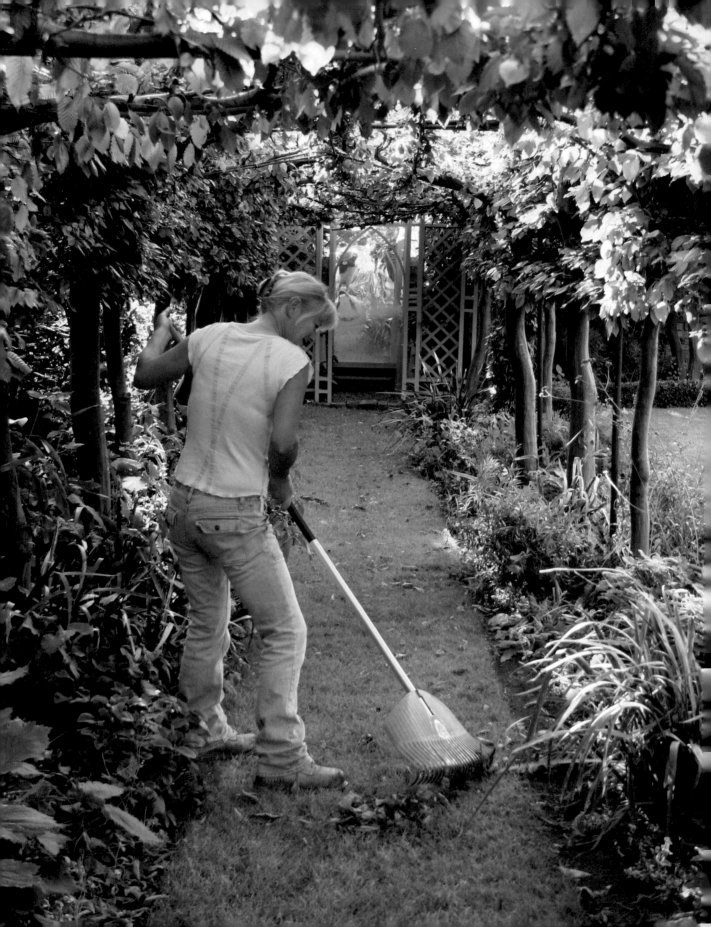

Dutch (Scuffle) Hoe

For keeping weeds down among vegetables and in borders, a Dutch hoe (also called a scuffle hoe) is invaluable. It has a sharp, flat blade that you use with a push-pull action, so that it just travels in and scuffles the very top layer of soil, slicing the weeds off from their roots as it goes. In just five minutes you can quickly whip through a significant area so that weed control becomes lighter and more satisfying work.

This hoe causes little disturbance to the worms, provided you work in the surface layer. In dry periods you will want to retain as much moisture in the soil as possible. (Although it was once believed that if you hoed just the top surface, you would develop a 'dry mulch' that would sit on the top and conserve the moisture below, this is now thought to be incorrect; any tillage of the soil surface in dry weather will cause moisture loss.) In damp periods, tenacious, disturbed weeds may regrow, so hoeing in the rain is often counterproductive. Keep your hoe sharpened with a sharpening stone—and to avoid leaving tracks in the garden, try walking backwards with it.

Draw Hoe

Although the draw hoe is more commonly found in gardens than the Dutch hoe is, the draw hoe is less useful. Its blade is positioned at a right angle to its shaft and it is helpful, although not essential, for the job of taking out drills when sowing seed. It is also used for chopping out odd clumps of weeds.

Rakes

The main varieties of rake include lawn rakes, leaf rakes, and soil or garden rakes. The latter is necessary for preparing a level seed bed and raking gravel. If you watch Japanese gardeners raking gravel to perfection, you realize that the process is as soothing to your mind as it is good, gentle exercise for the body. Just remember to rake in a balanced way, by alternating the arm you use to rake.

Hedge Cutters

The hedge cutter you choose will depend on the scale of the task for which it is needed. For more heavy-duty jobs (deciduous hedges in excess of 330 ft. or 100 m with tractor access) flail mowers (usually tractor-mounted) are indispensable but should only be used by experienced operators. If you have hedging of less than 330 ft. (100 m), you have a choice between electric, petrol, and battery-operated machines. Battery-operated machines will work for twenty to forty minutes before recharging, and are light and convenient. For lengths over 165 ft. (50 m), a petrol machine is most efficient, but heavier.

You will also need to decide whether you require a trimmer or a cutter. Trimmers have shorter teeth with smaller distances between them and produce a neater finish. Cutters have larger teeth with larger spacings and are good for chunkier growth, producing a more rugged finish.

Always try hedge cutters before purchasing to ensure that they are easy to handle. If you have high hedges, you can buy cordless trimmers with long-reach extensions; some can cut about 8 ft. (2.5 m) above your arm's reach. The blade can also be angled for cutting tops. For cutting low hedges, seek out a battery-operated mini trimmer that is light and easy to use from all angles.

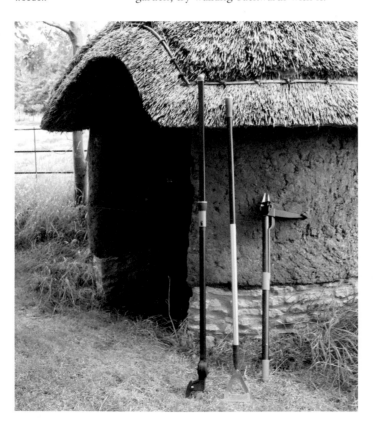

LEFT: This wide, long-handled leaf and lawn rake with big, flat teeth is easy to use and efficient to use.

BELOW (LEFT TO RIGHT): A long-reach pruner, a Dutch hoe, and a weeder.

Stocking Your Toolshed

MISCELLANEOUS TOOLS

So many specially designed ergonomic tools are on the market today that there is bound to be one that addresses your individual needs. This is a small sampling; see the Appendix for further resources.

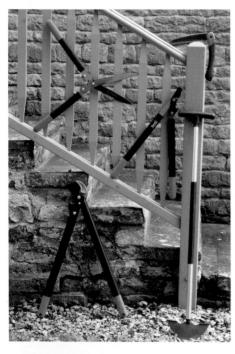

- If you do not like using ladders for high hedges, certain types of mechanical hedge cutters have lightweight telescopic extensions with angled heads.
- A flame gun with a gas cylinder will keep weeds at bay in gravelly areas without the need to bend or kneel over. The easiest ones to use are those that ignite automatically without the need for a lighter, allowing you to turn them on and off quickly. (Lighting them can be rather scary.) This method is quicker than hoeing and is useful for large areas of gravel. It is an organic alternative to chemical weed control.
- Deadheading, planting, and many more garden tasks involve kneeling. If you need help getting up and down when you kneel, go for a kneeler with handles. Some versions will fold up, making them easier to carry around and store. Some can also be turned upside down and used as seats.
- Cordless, lightweight clippers that are especially easy to handle will make the repetitive actions of clipping topiary less taxing on your hands and wrists.
- Tools with a non-slip grip provide greater control for gardeners with arthritic hands and fingers.

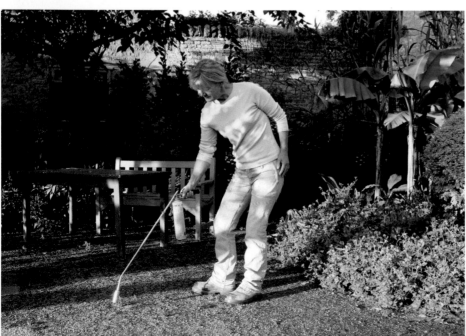

ABOVE LEFT (CLOCKWISE FROM TOP LEFT): hedge shears, a retractable pruning saw, medium bypass loppers, a long-handled edger, and large anvil loppers.

LEFT: A flame gun is an effective tool for weeding gravelly areas without the need to bend over.

Hand, Wrist, and Elbow Care

Many garden activities, such as trimming hedges, pruning shrubs, or planting bedding plants, cause you to use your hands in the same way over and over again as you grip your gardening tool. This sort of repetitive action can lead to a feeling of strain, particularly if your technique is not right; having excellent 'posture' in the garden does not apply exclusively to your body position, but also to your wrists.

Discomfort in the hands, wrists, and elbows relates to the entire body. It makes a big difference when you engage your shoulders as well as your deep stabilizing muscles rather than just your wrists and forearms in isolation. Visualize the movement originating from your shoulder girdle (your shoulder joint and your shoulder blade) and imagine your entire body as being centred.

Your grip strength is best when your wrist is in a relaxed or neutral position; if you bend your wrist, your wrist strength is reduced by up to 25%. Not only is the bent position less efficient, but it is also more hazardous: the tendons that flex the fingers are aggravated by movements made while your hand is assuming this position.

To avoid developing disorders like tendonitis and carpal tunnel syndrome, practise good gripping technique: do not bend your wrist when you grasp pruners and other hand tools, and imagine the movement stemming from your shoulders.

BELOW: Holding your wrist in its straight, neutral position in the garden will help protect you from strain and injury.

WRIST POSITION

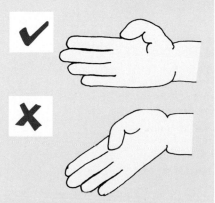

If your wrist is kept in a relatively neutral position (TOP), your muscle tendons are able to work as effectively as possible and very little stress is inflicted on your wrists. Contrastingly, if your wrist is held in a bent or distorted position (ABOVE), your muscle tendons could be placed under stress, as they have to turn a corner and are stretched. Gripping garden tools with your wrist in this position can lead to strain and should be avoided.

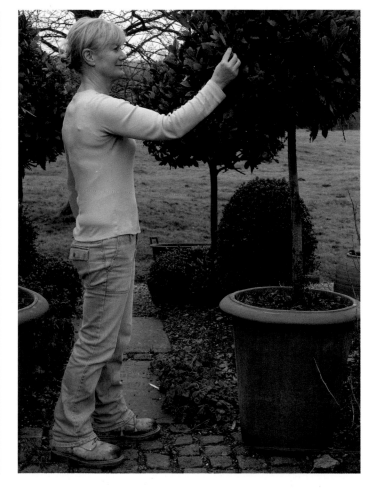

Hand, Wrist, and Elbow Care

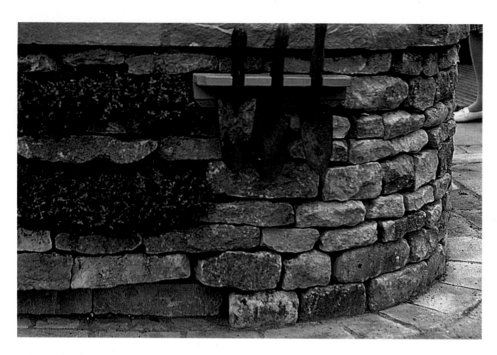

Many of us are prone to losing small hand trowels, so it is nice to own several at a time!

ERGONOMIC HAND TOOLS

Supplementing your basic tool shed with a few of the following tools will help you to garden in a more efficient and safe manner. The ones highlighted below are especially beneficial for minimizing the stress on the hands, wrists, and elbows.

Watering Cans and Barrels

Some watering cans are lightweight and have plastic extensions that twist so that you can water your plants without twisting your wrists. If this is too difficult, then some watering cans are designed to deliver a stream of water upon pressing a button and it is worth seeking these out.

To make watering quicker when using a can, place a large water barrel beside the tap and dunk your can into it whenever you need water, rather than waiting for the can to fill up.

Lightweight Shears

When you prune, lightweight shears are easier to use as they reduce the stress that is inflicted upon your wrists. Small, cordless, rechargeable hand trimmers are especially useful for intricate work.

Finger Grips

Many tools come with moulded finger grips on the handles for extra grip strength. A drawback is that they only fit one size of hand perfectly; if your hands are larger, your fingers will overlap the grooves uncomfortably, causing calluses and soreness, while smaller hands will have to stretch awkwardly, which reduces the grip strength and so requires more pressure to maintain control of the tool.

Hand Tools for Special Needs

If you have problems with one or both wrists, specially designed hand tools are available. These hand tools have angled (vertical) handles that render them far more comfortable to use. By ensuring that your hand and wrist are positioned at a natural angle (see diagram on page 87), these tools help to eliminate the stresses that can be inflicted by conventionally styled tools. Add-on handles an also be attached to regular hand tools—and larger grips, or even a piece of foam wrapped around the tool's handle, can also provide an easier grip for sufferers of arthritis. (PETA supplies these tools; for more information, see Appendix.)

Hand Trowel

A hand trowel lets you indulge in close cultivation, allowing you to get very close to the soil surface and, of course, to your plants. There is huge variability in price; whether you go for a cheaper model because you frequently mislay them or invest in the top of the range is up to you.

Some gardeners prefer a pointed end to the blade, which allows for more intricate work. Quite a few are partial to the stainless steel variety which does not generally become clogged up with soil. Because you will use a trowel often, spoil yourself and get both a large-scoop, broad trowel and a narrow one with a serrated edge that cuts through soil more easily. You may want to fit a wrist strap onto your hand trowel which will make the action less strenuous on your wrists. To avoid overclenching your fist, make sure that the size of your trowel's grips fits your hand. If you have have pain in your hand joints, a handle with a large diameter or a contoured grip will make the trowel easier to use. A long-handled trowel will help you to avoid overreaching.

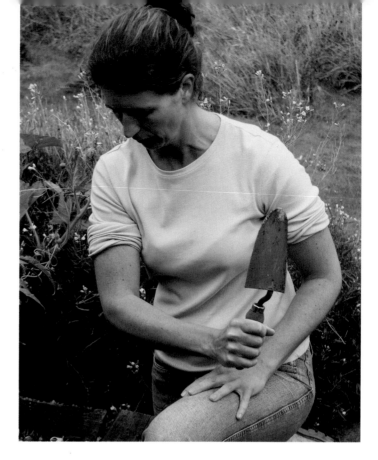

When a hand tool is grasped too hard, visible tension is generated in the neck, wrist, and forearm.

TENNIS ELBOW: A COMMON GARDENER'S COMPLAINT

If you feel pain and tenderness in the outer part of your elbow that worsens when you extend your wrist against resistance, it is likely that you suffer from lateral epicondylitis, which is known as tennis elbow. This condition usually stems from the overuse of muscles located in your forearms which pull your hands backwards when you carry out any repetitive movement involving a grip. These forearm muscles, known as wrist extensors, insert into the bony protuberance just above your elbow, which is called the lateral epicondyle. Because the bony protuberance into which the muscles insert has a small surface area, the forces generated when you grip something repetitively can place stress on the lateral epicondyle, setting up an inflammatory response that is felt in the outer elbow.

In the garden, repetitive gripping actions such as hedge trimming or digging can stress the wrist extensors and bring about tennis elbow. This condition can be treated through mobilization, acupuncture, or steroid injection, and sometimes a brace can be worn on the forearm, which helps to alleviate the forces that are placed on the bone. If you believe that you have this condition, you must seek medical advice from a doctor or a physiotherapist.

However, this uncomfortable condition is largely preventable. Changing your gardening technique can really help to prevent tennis elbow. The key is to choose a tool with a hand grip that is the right size for you, which helps to avoid gripping too hard and overclenching while carrying out repetitive movements.

Foot Care

Like the spine, feet have their own neutral stance position. Think of each foot as a tripod; it works best when your body weight is evenly distributed among your big toe, your little toe, and your heel. When your feet are in neutral, the muscles in your feet draw your toes back towards the heel without curling them, maintaining your foot's medial arch. Wearing sturdy shoes or boots that offer good arch support will help to hold your feet in their neutral position as you move through the garden. They lift your arches and prevent them from collapsing inwards.

Some people (for instance, ballet dancers who have been trained to go up *en pointe*) will have naturally high arches and therefore will not need medial arch support, as their muscles will manage to keep their feet in place. However, the vast majority of us have a tendency towards flat feet or dropped arches. It is important to make sure that your footwear has adequate arch support. Most gardeners need a pair of warm and

waterproof boots for colder, wetter weather in addition to a pair of comfortable shoes that work well when it is hot and sunny.

WELLINGTON BOOTS

Wellington boots used to be the preserve of the English, but now their popularity is spreading around the world. Huge advances have been made in materials, so that these boots are no longer sweaty, stiff, and uncomfortable like they once were.

A major advantage of Wellington boots is they are easy to slip on and off. If these are your gardening footwear of choice, it is worth investing in a good pair. Even the most expensive are good value when you compare the price with that of more fashionable, non-gardening boots. You will wear your gardening boots for many years and if they keep your feet feeling great, then they are really not an unforgivable extravagance.

Choose your liner carefully. The most sophisticated Wellingtons have linings

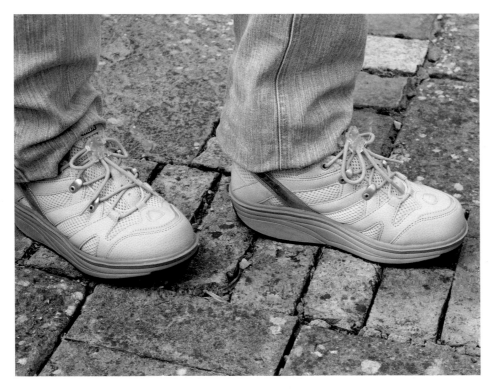

These Masai Barefoot Technology shoes have curved soles which may encourage some people to find neutral alignment and improve their posture and balance. Using these shoes correctly requires concentration; if you are used to standing with your back either flat or overarched, then you may initially find them challenging to wear.

with a material called Outlast, originally developed by NASA for astronauts, which has the ability to draw excess heat away from the feet when hot, and releases it back when they are cold; when you put your feet in them on a warm day, you really notice the difference. For perennially cold feet, Neoprene is a snug liner that many Wellington boot manufacturers now use. It is a superb insulator and also provides lots of cushioning, so it puts real spring in your step. It is especially helpful if you have a bad back, as it reduces jarring on an uneven surface.

If you have large calves, or like a really shapely fit, you should choose boots with a gusset in the side so when you have tucked in your jeans you are not restricting the blood flow to your lower legs.

Another useful feature is a strengthened sole. A good sole is important to support the foot in its neutral position. Many of z Aigle range (see Appendix) feature stiffened midsoles so that they last longer with continuous digging. Many manufacturers also make shorter Wellingtons, which some gardeners find more comfortable as well.

OTHER BOOTS

If you prefer an ankle-type boot with laces, choose one with an insulated sole, as well as a not-too-rigid feel (so that you can move your feet around). Some are quite heavy too, which you really notice by the end of the day; unless you want to focus on building up muscle tone, these are best avoided.

SHOES FOR LIGHTER WORK

For lighter summer work, you can choose from a wider variety of garden shoes that are often more attractive and fun to wear than their hardier cold-weather counterparts. Garden clogs are common, as are espadrilles and even flip-flops. Certain companies offer designated gardening shoes; for instance, Muckboot (who make colourful and functional Wellingtons) also make a garden shoe called The Eden. It is comfortable, waterproof and easy to slip on and off, and works with shorts, jeans, or a skirt. Trainers (or sneakers) can also work well for lighter gardening and allow you to move seamlessly between gardening and supplementary aerobic exercise such as jogging.

FIRST AID FOR MINOR INJURIES

Injuries cannot always be prevented and sometimes accidents happen. If you are injured in the garden, or suffer from recurrent strain, you should seek professional medical advice from a doctor or chartered physiotherapist—particularly if you have any open wound, suspect a fracture, or sustain any injury that does not improve in 48 hours. It helps to write down what happened and how it occurred so that you have a record of the date and time of onset as well as the mechanism of injury when you seek help.

Self-diagnosis can be very difficult unless the injury has happened before, and even then it can be unreliable. The advice given in this chapter applies only to minor injuries and is no substitute for medical guidance.

If you suspect a sprained muscle, you can deliver first aid by following the **PRICE** regime:

Protect the injured part from further damage by ensuring that the surrounding area is safe.

Rest the injured part. Try to keep it as still as possible.

Ice the injury. This is done in order to limit bleeding.

Compression will help to reduce swelling. Apply firm bandages or compression splints, making sure that they are not so tight that they impede circulation.

Elevation of the injured part will help to prevent further swelling and aid in recovery.

The affected body part should be positioned so that it is higher than the heart in order to aid venous return (the return of fluid to the heart). Resting an injured arm, leg, or other part of the body on a stack of pillows works well; if a lower limb is injured, this will involve lying down.

Choosing Your Mower

The process of choosing a mower deserves special attention as it is a leading source of confusion among gardeners. Mowers are expensive pieces of equipment, and they can vary tremendously when it comes to both efficiency and conduciveness to health and fitness.

The type of finish required, coupled with the amount of time and exertion you want to expend, will determine which mower is right for you. To decide which machine will suit you best, it is important to go to a reputable dealer and try a wide range of different models. Some of the most popular mowers are highlighted on the right.

Do not forget that mown grass is one of the most expensive garden surfaces in terms of hours needed to tend it throughout the year. As grass is relatively inexpensive to establish, we conveniently tend to forget this!

You can, of course, reduce the mowing frequency of some grass, and cut it quite high (to 4 in. [10 cm] or so). This will reduce the vigour of the grass, and save you time—but it is only an option if your mower is capable of cutting and collecting or mulching at longer lengths. There are other time-saving options as well—but having the right equipment to cut your grass is the key.

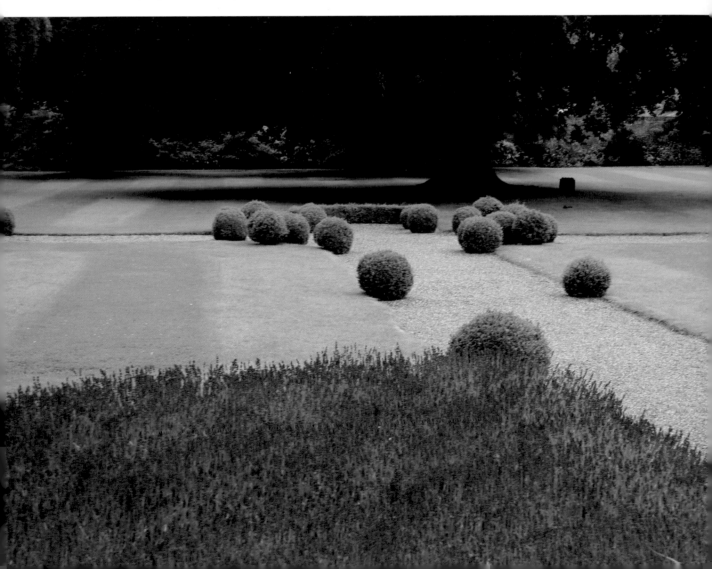

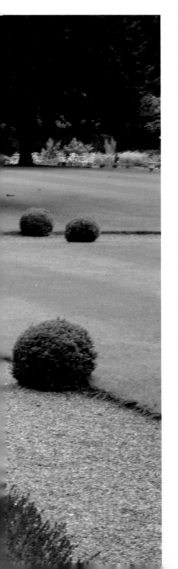

To achieve this pristine (and very high-maintenance) finish, you will need to use a cylinder (reel) mower on a level lawn.

MOWER COMPARISON CHART

MOWER STYLE	AREA/HR	CALORIES/HR
Cylinder (Reel) (18 in./45 cm)	1/3 acre	250

Requires that you cut more frequently, often twice weekly in rapid growing times, as you can only cut around 1/2 in. (12 mm) at a time. Can be time-consuming, as you may need to empty cuttings from the mower's box; for this, allow another half hour per 1/3 acre.

Engineless Cylinder (14 in./35 cm)	200 square yards	340

Only suitable for postage-stamp-sized areas, but a 'green' machine that is great exercise, with no noise and no awkward engine.

Rotary (18 in./45 cm)	1/3 acre	250

Allows you to leave a longer interval between cuts than you can with a cylinder (reel) mower because it can cope with cutting longer grass. Again, if you collect the cuttings you'll need to spend another half hour emptying the box per hour spent mowing.

Mulching (18 in./45 cm)	1/3 acre	250

Spares you the task of collecting grass; on the other hand, you will need to mow more frequently in rapid growing times.

Ride-on (Riding) (38 in./105 cm)	1 acre	140

Affords you almost no physical exercise, saves time only when mowing large expanses of grass, and is typically the most expensive kind of mower. A ride-on (riding) mower cannot tackle smaller patches of grass so you may need to buy an additional, smaller mower as well. You may need to factor in significant extra time for emptying the box.

Ride-on Mulching (see above)	1 acre	140

May require that you mow more frequently in rapid growing periods. The comments above apply, but it is faster than a traditional ride-on (riding) mower as you will not need to empty its box.

Hand-held Strimmer with Cord	1/4 acre	340

Requires you to rake up too, which is good exercise but is time-consuming; factor in 30 minutes of raking per 1/4 acre cut.

Hover Mower (18 in./45 cm)	1/3 acre	225

Often requires that you collect grass cuttings, as the hover mower's built-in collection system can be inefficient.

Choosing Your Mower

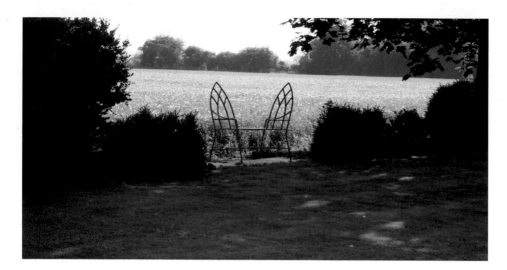

LEFT: By borrowing some space from 'next door', this grassy part of the garden appears more expansive. Cultivating a weed-free lawn next to this field will be a struggle, though, as weed seeds will always encroach.

THE CYLINDER (REEL) MOWER: FOR HIGH-MAINTENANCE LAWNS

If you want a 'stripe' on your lawn and a top-notch finish, a cylinder (reel) mower will be your best option. As precision-made pieces of equipment, cylinder (reel) mowers are often expensive: they typically cost one-and-a-half times as much rotary mowers do, and their servicing costs tend to be more than double. You need an almost pancake-flat lawn to enable it to function well, but you do get an amazing finish.

A cylinder (reel) mower is the essential accessory for a high-maintenance lawn. Mowing twice a week with a this mower will be necessary in order to keep your grass looking trim during times of the year when growth is particularly rapid. Some gardeners leave the collecting box permanently off, to build up humus levels; the front-mounted collecting box limits the mower's manoeuvering potential. If you notice that the mower is failing to cut the longer flower stalks, it is probably due to blades that have become blunt and need sharpening.

THE ROTARY MOWER: DESERVEDLY POPULAR

Rotary mowers are easy to use and are the most popular utilitarian mower, although mulching mowers are rapidly catching up. Some rotaries will produce a fairly decent stripe on your lawn. The rear-mounted box is easier to manoeuvre, and with the box off, the clippings shoot out of the back to form an orderly line in the mower's wake. (With a cylinder [reel] mower, contrastingly, the cuttings fly everywhere, into neighbouring pools, beds and sand pits.)

Make sure that you keep the blades of your rotary mower sharp. Examine the grass two days after cutting: if the leaves are white at their ends and jagged and bent over at their tips, this means that the blades need sharpening. Keeping an extra set of blades on hand will ensure that your mower is never out of action.

THE RIDE-ON (RIDING) MOWER: LEAST PHYSICALLY DEMANDING

Using a ride-on (riding) mower is not good exercise! If you have less than half an acre of grass and are physically adept enough to push a mower, do not resort to a riding mower as it often will not save you any time at all.

Moreover, these mowers tend to cost more than other mowers—factor in not just initial financial outlay, but also servicing (including collection) and fuel which are all far more expensive than that of the other mowers. You will often need to purchase an additional smaller mower to tackle smaller grassy areas. What's more, the time you spend mowing will not be significantly reduced until you get into beefier areas.

RIGHT: This grass edge was made by retaining the newly sown grass edge with a timber board for a few months. Once the grass had established the board was removed, leaving the lawn 2 in. (5 cm) proud of the path. The cylinder mower is then able to cut right to the edge with no risk of damage to the blades.

THE HOVER MOWER:
FOR A ROUGHER FINISH

Hover mowers are certainly not for perfectionists; the finish you get from these lightweight, and often very inexpensive, mowers will not be very high-quality, and they will not leave a stripe on your lawn. Typically, hover mowers will cut down to under ½ in. (1.5 cm), but will not cut grass that is any higher than about 3 in. (7 cm) and so are not advisable for areas with longer grass. On a positive note, they are useful for banks and can target slopes of up to 45° (petrol) or slightly greater (electric). An extra-lightweight version with plastic blades is a clever option for older gardeners or anyone who finds the regular version uncomfortable to wield for longer periods.

THE MULCHING MOWER:
EASY AND EFFICIENT

Mulching mowers are excellent for busy people who want to get the job done well in a shorter amount of time. With a mulching mower there is no need to pick up cuttings, which massively reduces the amount of time you need to spend mowing.

These machines shred up the clippings into pieces the size of a tea leaf (twenty times smaller than the average clipping), returning them back to the lawn, which continuously improves the structure of the soil. This is especially helpful during dry summers and on thin soils, as it helps to keep the grass green when it would otherwise dry out. During times of rapid growth, it will be necessary to cut the lawn once every four to seven days, and if you miss a cut or two, you will need to go over it two times or more (but never collecting the mowings) to create a 'respectable' finish.

You should never cut more than a third of the length off at a time, and it is vital to keep the underside of the cutting deck clean. A simple way to do this is to spray it with dashboard cleaner (a silicone spray). Some of these mowers will produce a stripe of sorts, but it will not compete with that of a cylinder (reel) mower. Contrary to popular belief, mulching mowers do not usually cause a build up of thatch, and the shredded cuttings do not get stuck to shoes. For gardeners who want an easy, efficient tool for attaining a neat lawn, these mowers take a lot of beating.

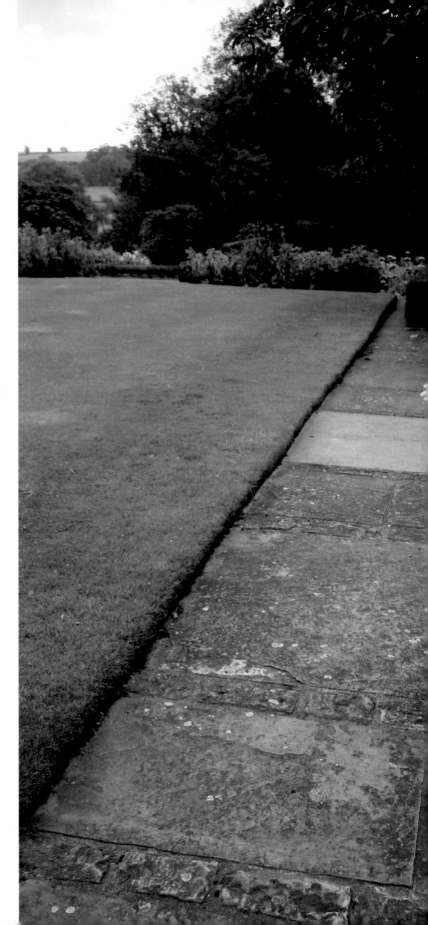

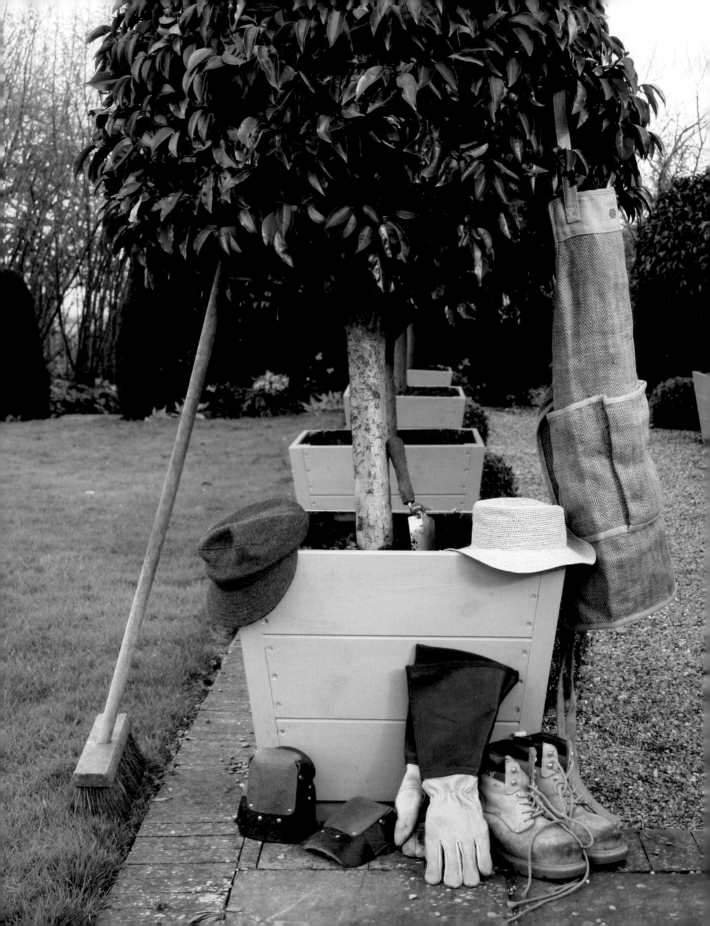

Protection from the Elements

The following accessories will make your life easier in the garden.

GLOVES

Prolonged exposure to soil, water, and ultraviolet rays really ages gardeners' hands before their time; sadly, most gardeners are recognizable by the state of their hands, which often resemble tortoise feet even in their early years. Donning gardening gloves will protect hands from the elements. If you can find gloves that suit you and get into the habit of wearing them whenever you garden, the protection they afford saves endless delving for splinters, application of moisturizing creams, and cleaning nails.

Gloves that are too thick or very loose will affect your grip because they cause your fingers to spread too far apart. Even cotton gloves will reduce your grip strength by about 25%. Very thin gloves, on the other hand, can feel like a second skin and allow for very intricate work. The latex-style gloves worn by doctors and dentists for examinations are ideal. A downside is that these gloves are essentially disposable—you may go through a pair or two each day—so if you are concerned about sustainability you may prefer to use traditional, thicker gloves. (However, you might think of your thin, disposable gloves as a forgivable extravagance, as they let you work in the garden with great precision, while doing a great job of protecting your hands.)

Natural latex can occasionally cause an allergic reaction where the skin becomes irritated and itchy in patches. To be safe, it is best to choose latex-style gloves that are made of synthetic materials such as rubber, nitrile, vinyl, or neoprene.

For working in warm weather, where you do not need such precision but you still want a second-skin feel, you can find hard-wearing, washable nitrile gloves that come in three sizes and bright colours (see Appendix). Many professionals swear by these gloves, as they are ideal for most jobs except pricking out seedlings and sowing seeds. When it is cold and wet, latex gloves can be worn underneath to make them waterproof and increase the insulation. For quite intricate work in wintry or wet conditions, a good solution is a thin silk or wool glove with a heavy-duty, fairly close-fitting rubber glove over the top.

GAUNTLETS

When you are pulling out thistles and nettles in long grass or struggling with brambles and ramblers, heavy-duty gauntlets (gloves that cover your forearms, as well as your hands) will allow you to delve in deeper with less wear and tear on your hands and arms. It is worth investing in a high-quality pair, especially if you have wilder and slightly overgrown spaces in your garden; even though you will not use your gauntlets every day, they can make the management of these more overgrown spaces considerably less taxing.

APRONS

Quickly slipping an apron over your clothes lets you dash out into the garden at any time, regardless of what you are wearing. A spontaneous decision to water a plant or pick some spinach can often lead to prolonged forays in the garden, and the apron will protect your 'proper' clothes from becoming soiled as you get your hands dirty. Try to choose one with pockets for garden tools.

HATS

Hats are more than mere cosmetic frippery; for protection against skin cancer and the aging effects of the sun, hats with wide brims and peaks give essential protection against ultraviolet rays.

The ideal gardening hat should be comfortable, and it should fit snugly enough to stay on even when the wind is gusting. Indulge in a selection for different temperatures, rain, and shine and get into the habit of regularly wearing one, along with high-protection-factor face cream, even if you are only planning to spend a few minutes gardening. After all, as most keen gardeners know, five minutes working in the sunshine can easily turn into an hour!

LEFT (CLOCKWISE FROM TOP RIGHT): A hand trowel, a rustic apron, a straw hat for warmer weather, boots with insulated soles and steel toecaps, gauntlets, sturdy and comfortable knee pads, a Baker Boy hat for winter wear, and a broom.

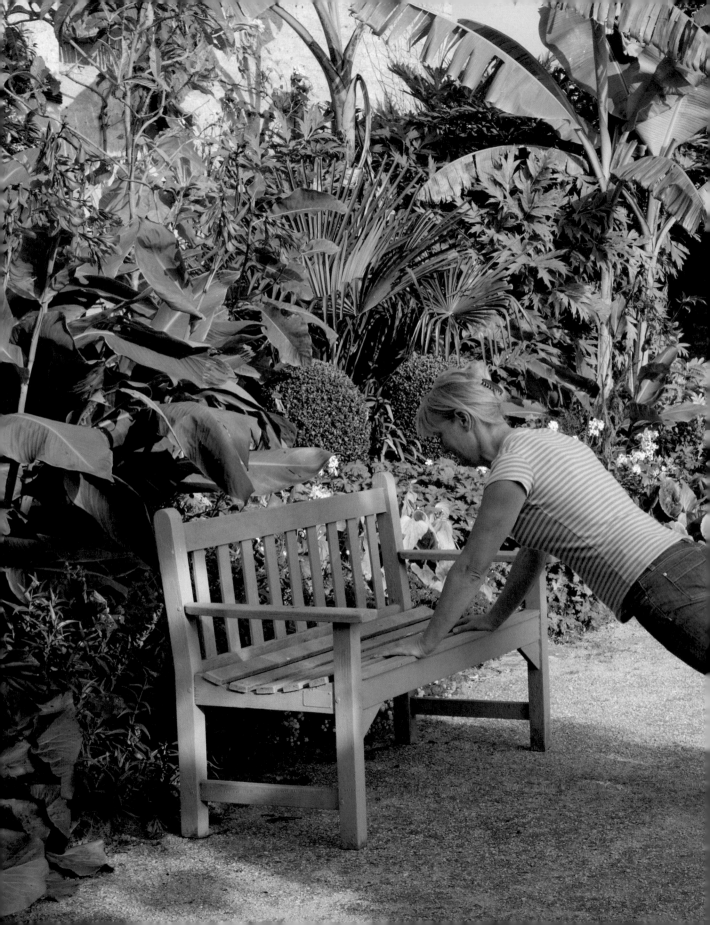

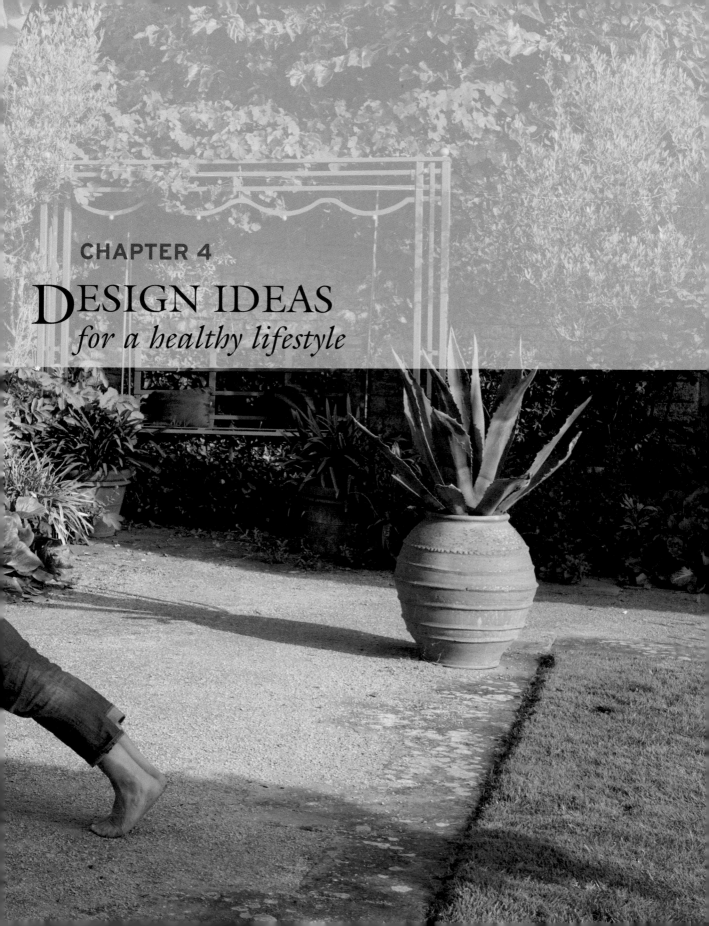

CHAPTER 4

DESIGN IDEAS
for a healthy lifestyle

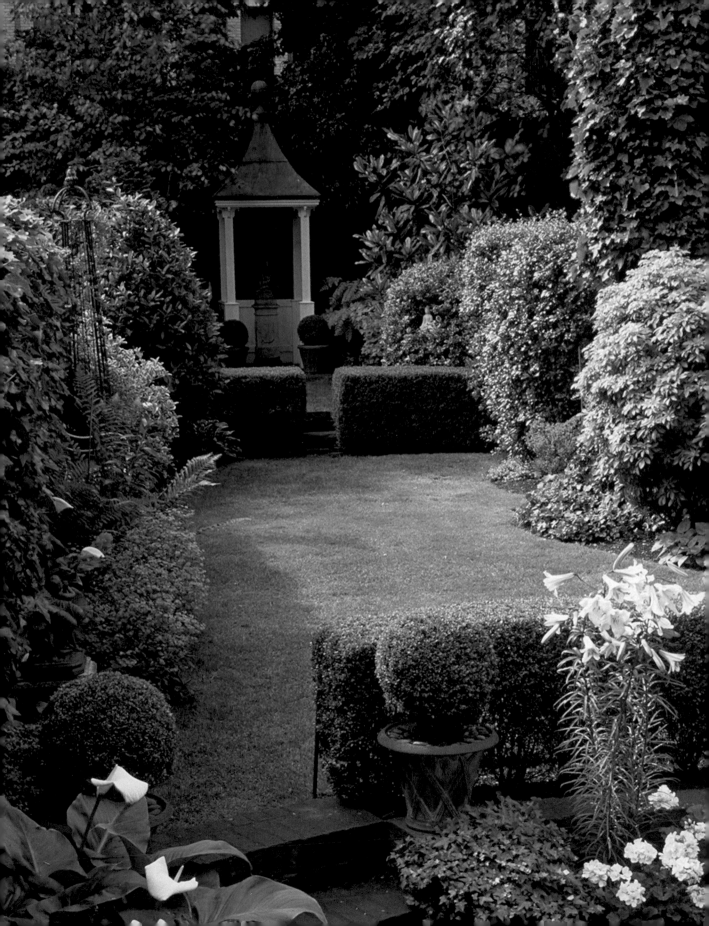

WITH CAREFUL design and clever use of landscaping materials, it is possible to create a garden that complements your healthy lifestyle superbly. Regardless of how big or small it is, your garden should be designed in a way that brings out its versatility and liveability. It should encourage you to stay active while also offering soothing, enticing spaces for relaxation and enjoyment.

Some gardeners dabble with their space and then become frustrated when it never measures up to their expectations. For best results (and peace of mind), it is worth taking the time to craft a 'master plan' for your garden which you can implement over the years by planting shelterbelts, building trim trails, putting in hedges for privacy, implementing borders (whether they are extravagantly high-maintenance, or simple enough that they virtually care for themselves), adding paving areas or lawns to serve as outdoor gyms, and so on. The plan will hopefully keep you on the right track and allow you to proceed with its implementation at a rate that suits you, whether your plans come to fruition in one season or over a decade or more.

If young children can be encouraged to use the outdoor space, this gets them into the habit of exploring and enjoying the outdoor environment, and they can build on that inclination for the rest of their lives. Then, a few years later (when those children leave home and you have more free time), a stimulating garden can really come into its own. If you develop a strong structure, your garden can literally grow into it and the various spaces can be adapted to cater for the needs of the different people who will be using it. Gardens are dynamic and ever-changing places that can be tailormade to suit our tastes, support our fitness goals, and inspire wellbeing—and despite our best-laid plans, they always surprise us.

Try to design inviting spaces to cater for different activities. Entertaining, relaxing, playing, exercising, and (of course) gardening are all accommodated in this relatively compact garden.

A Plan for Health and Wellbeing

Whether you are creating a new garden from scratch, revamping one that already exists, or hoping to add a few minor touches that will promote health and wellbeing, sitting down to sketch a plan for your garden is an extremely useful process. In addition to giving you a sense of how the different elements of your garden fit together, it will help you understand what will (and will not) be possible to achieve in your particular outdoor space.

When planning the design of your garden, using an accurately scaled survey helps tremendously. It may be possible to undertake the survey yourself, possibly based on a site-centred Ordnance Survey plan (in England) or the U.S. Geological Survey (in the United States). These can be altered to a convenient scale and used as a base plan. By using two long measuring tapes, you can obtain all of the additional information, such as the position of trees, paths, and borders, that is required in order to draw up a complete survey plan to a given scale. There are a number of books that explain this process in detail.

If you find this daunting, or your garden is too large or complex, you can employ a professional surveyor to carry out the survey of your property and generate a scaled drawing of it for you, complete with precise dimensions, levels, and angles. Gardeners who commission these surveys are often very surprised when they receive the scaled plan of their garden from the surveyor, as the relative sizes of different areas often deviate wildly from what they had expected.

The next step is to compose a (realistic) wish list of all the features that you covet. These may include a play area, a lawn, a wildlife pool, or a treehouse—the possibilities are endless. It may be that you cannot afford or do not have the time to put into place what you want at first, but it is worth earmarking spaces for everything you hope to include in your garden so that they can be accommodated in the future. For instance, if a large paved area is beyond your budget at the present time, you could gravel this space initially and use just a few slabs. This would allow you to establish the framework of planting around it immediately.

Having obtained your survey and finalized your wish list, you can experiment with tracing paper overlays, trying out

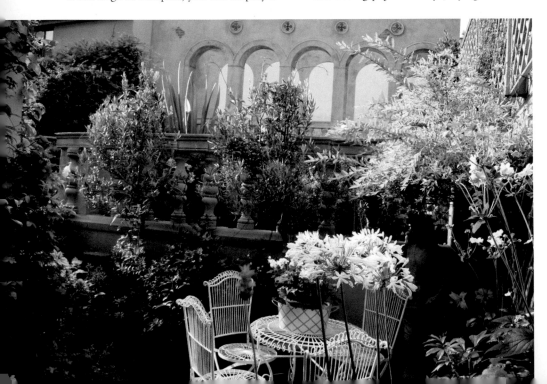

This garden was previously dominated by an ugly garage with a flat roof. To conceal it, the wall was rendered and a *trompe l'oeil* was painted over it. A slope was altered to create three distinct and useable levels.

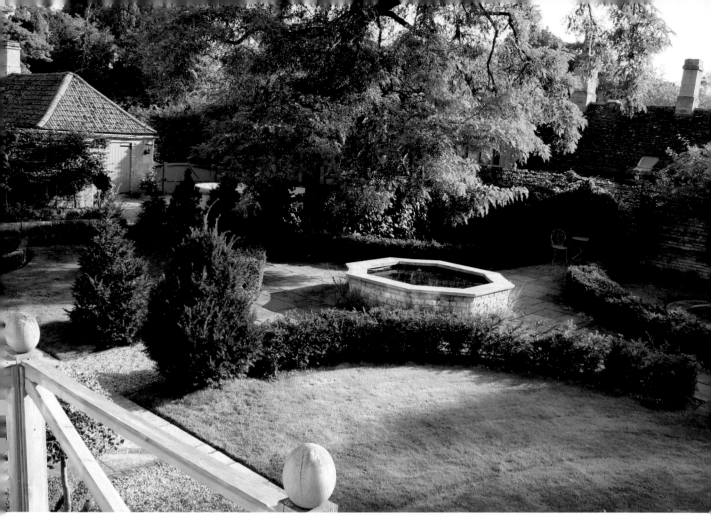

This garden was designed for two energetic young boys and their keen gardening parents. A large, sunken trampoline is tucked away to the right, the treehouse is up in the central tree, and the bright blue swimming pool is just barely visible in the top left corner.

different design permutations. This part is not easy, especially if you are unfamiliar with plans, scales, and design.

It may save you many frustrating years if you consult help from a professional landscape architect or garden designer. However, you should first be sure to have a look at other gardens they have worked on to decide whether you like their approach.

When planning a garden that supports your health and fitness goals, the following considerations are often neglected, but deserve special attention.

1. CONSIDER THE RELATIONSHIP BETWEEN GARDEN AND HOUSE

Certain parts of the garden—particularly the area near the entrance and the main views from the house—are on view nearly all of the time. These areas need to be designed and planted so that their 'on' periods are as long as possible (and their 'off' periods as short as possible).

By virtue of their prominent position, these areas are often more highly structured than other parts of the garden, and it is usually worthwhile to lavish a bit more time and effort upon these high-profile spots.

Looking at a fabulous garden has a habit of bringing about both tranquility and stimulation, and making attractive features visible from the house will encourage you to walk through your garden, enjoy it, and exercise in it. To this end, when carrying out building alterations or additions, it is vital that you carefully consider elements such as access points (entrances should be easy to use) and windowsill heights (ideally they should be low enough to let you view the garden when sitting down). Pay close attention to positions of French doors, and locations of studies, sinks, and kitchens. To glimpse copious foliage, colourful flowers, and moving boughs from inside and from the area around your house allows you to enjoy these features to their fullest.

If your garden of vegetables and herbs is easily accessible from your kitchen door, you will most likely find time to snatch a few herbs for most meals—something fresh, fast, and healthy. If your garden tools hang just a few strides from the kitchen door, you will probably be more inclined to deadhead a rose or remove the odd weed while waiting for a phone call or for the kettle to boil. Sometimes it works the other way, however; placing your greenhouse a brisk walk away from your kitchen will compel you to walk in the fresh air whenever you need to go there, and will make the greenhouse seem like a private haven, removed from the house—affording you space to clear your thoughts while you mist your cuttings or open and shut the doors.

2. ADDRESS PROBLEMS

While you are trying out different garden layouts on the tracing overlays, make sure that you address any elements of the garden that you consider to be problematic. Common 'problems' include overlooking neighbours, noise from external sources, ugly views of immovable objects, or undesirable aspects of the house such as

unsightly additions or bleak walls. Once you have analyzed these flaws, make sure that your design counteracts them as much as possible.

Try to make the most of the available space so that it is really useable and addresses your needs. For instance, you may have a lovely paved area just outside your kitchen door, which in an ideal world would be perfect for aerobic exercise routines—if it were not battered by southwesterly winds and overlooked. By planting a hedge and a row of pleached trees in the vicinity, you can create a more sheltered, private space so that you will be able to exercise in this area with a measure of privacy, and without your mat and hair being continually swept away by the wind.

3. THINK CAREFULLY ABOUT MAINTENANCE LEVELS

Garden maintenance should be an opportunity to enjoy your garden while staying active, rather than a source of frustration. The amount of maintenance you are prepared to lavish upon your garden will influence its design. Being realistic about this will ensure that you do not suffer

This stone seat forms a resting place halfway up a flight of steps. The bank is densely planted with chamomile, and a rosemary hedge contains the informal planting behind. Chamomile lawns smell divine and require no mowing, but they tend to become gappy.

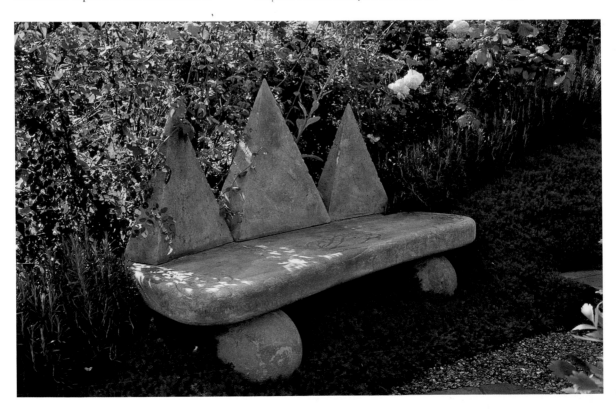

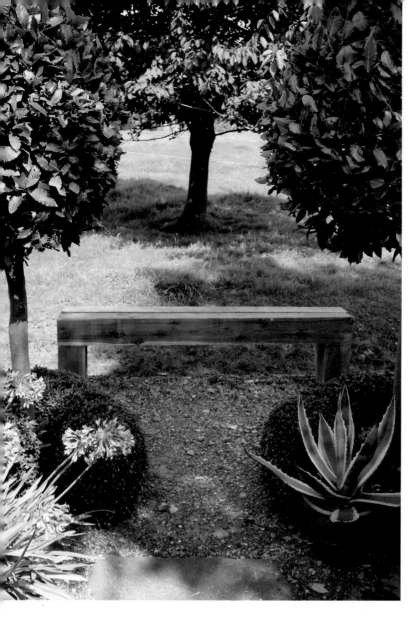

This small exercise bench doubles as a resting place. It was made from chunky pieces of timber fixed together.

forever). Lower-maintenance spaces need not be second best; they can be highly invigorating, injecting a relaxed, easygoing, and uncluttered feel into the garden. Try to introduce some understated 'wow factor' that really strikes a chord.

Often the maintenance burden of certain areas can be reduced by reconsidering the style you are aiming for. For instance, while pristine mown lawns are fabulous surfaces on which to run, play games, or sunbathe, they also demand to be cut on a regular basis—something a gym will not do! Leaving areas to be cut less frequently can make your lawn's maintenance far less demanding.

If you are space rich and time poor, a sound approach is to make the space look more natural. Many natural-looking planting styles look good most of the time; native woodland looks fabulous in all seasons, as do many meadows and less intensive orchards. Although they sound extensive and large-scale, miniature versions can be designed. Just a 2- or 3-yard (2- or 3-m) wide band of native-style trees will have room for an attractive understorey of ferns and wildflowers, and will have many of the visual qualities of a woodland. If you can widen it out in places it will then have the capacity to absorb a bench, swing, or log store. At the same time, it could screen an adjacent eyesore, provide shelter from winds, and pull in wildlife. By adding simple structure in the form of a green oak arch, a snaking path, or some funky sculpture, you can up the interest without committing to weeks of edging and trimming work.

Large pools or very simple bodies of water inevitably tend to have mesmerizing qualities. They often take significant time and effort to set up, but once installed they will not commit you to hours on your hands and knees. They can be fabulous spots for inducing tranquility and providing inspiration.

Keep in mind that your garden will grow with you. Like a young child, a garden is inevitably more demanding at first, but when it gets into its stride—that is, when the new plantings become established, weedy soils are cleaned up, and the bulk of your new projects have been accomplished—it becomes easier to fine-tune the maintenance demands to suit your lifestyle.

aggravation during frenetic times of the year when everything seems to be on the move.

High-maintenance gardens have their advantages; in the health and fitness sense, they keep you on your toes and an intensive maintenance burden can keep you active and focused on your fitness regime. However, if you aim for a clean, slick approach to design and maintenance, the sleek look will be eroded if the outlines of the hedges become blurred, the lawn invaded by weeds and moss, and the paving weathered by algae.

If in contrast you choose to cultivate a more relaxed, bohemian-style garden, certain maintenance tasks can generally be put on hold a bit longer (or, in some cases

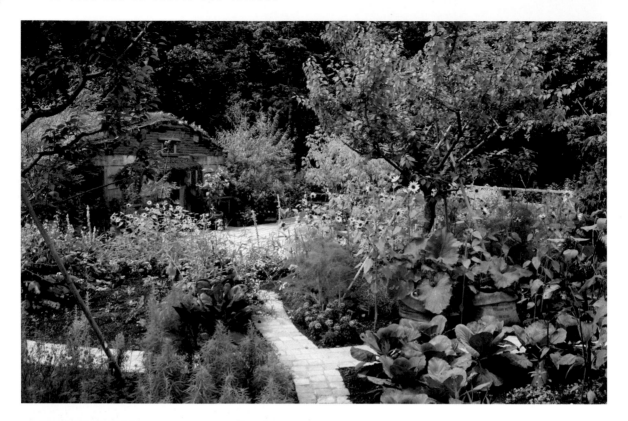

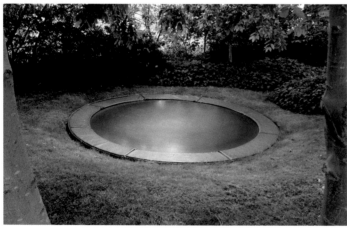

ABOVE: **This productive vegetable plot is sited in front of a playhouse for children. Small-scale paths around the beds provide an enticing area for games and the mix of tasty vegetables and bright flowers forms a colourful and stimulating backdrop.**

LEFT: **A few minutes spent jumping on a trampoline will burn calories, develop core strength, and improve balance and coordination. Sinking a trampoline into the ground minimizes its visual impact and makes it safer to use.**

4. CREATE SPACES FOR EXERCISE AND RELAXATION

In addition to creating an aesthetically pleasing space, you can also design a garden with distinct areas set aside for physical fitness. You may want to designate a surface for exercise, whether paved, gravel, on a mown lawn, or sheltered by trees in a woodland setting. Young families in particular can benefit hugely from having outdoor spaces devoted to games,

adventurous play and exercise right on their doorstep; fun outdoor spaces invite children to spend more time being active, rather than watching television.

In a more informal part of the garden, you may choose to create a trim trail. Even in smaller gardens, you can create a path network that will encourage you to jog or stroll around the garden. You can also incorporate steps for doing step-ups and banks for running up and down.

If your garden is on the compact side, you will need to be creative. A sunken trampoline, for instance, can be tucked away in a small space so that it is virtually invisible (and just ten minutes bouncing on it will burn quite a few calories). Another excellent option is to incorporate a horizontal beam beside a treehouse or climbing frame to provide a great framework for developing upper body muscles.

Bring out the liveability of your space. Designing in large paved surfaces with chairs and tables in readily accessible places such as right beside your kitchen window will encourage you to sit outside for that quick chat, cup of tea, or skim of the paper. Once you have ventured outside in the fresh air you may feel inclined to linger and do some gentle breathing exercises, or even the odd press-up on a nearby bench.

RIGHT: **A white garden seat looks special all year round; the holly that frames it requires just one annual cut.**

BELOW RIGHT: **This stylish yet very low-maintenance space, designed by Cleve West, has a great deal of impact and its bound gravel surface is both attractive and functional.**

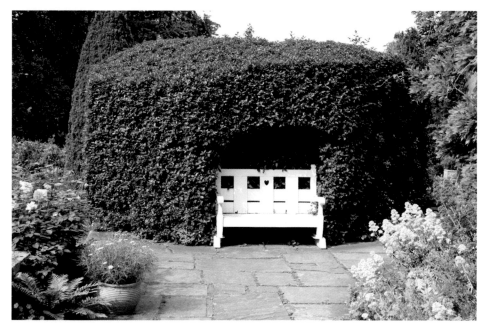

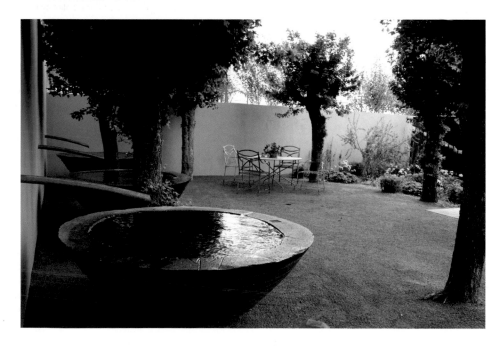

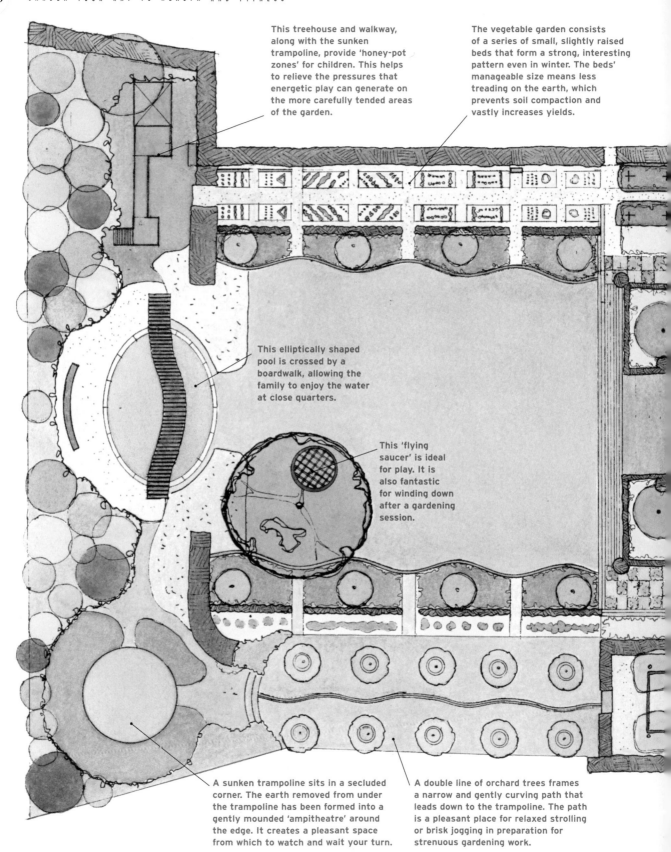

This treehouse and walkway, along with the sunken trampoline, provide 'honey-pot zones' for children. This helps to relieve the pressures that energetic play can generate on the more carefully tended areas of the garden.

The vegetable garden consists of a series of small, slightly raised beds that form a strong, interesting pattern even in winter. The beds' manageable size means less treading on the earth, which prevents soil compaction and vastly increases yields.

This elliptically shaped pool is crossed by a boardwalk, allowing the family to enjoy the water at close quarters.

This 'flying saucer' is ideal for play. It is also fantastic for winding down after a gardening session.

A sunken trampoline sits in a secluded corner. The earth removed from under the trampoline has been formed into a gently mounded 'ampitheatre' around the edge. It creates a pleasant space from which to watch and wait your turn.

A double line of orchard trees frames a narrow and gently curving path that leads down to the trampoline. The path is a pleasant place for relaxed strolling or brisk jogging in preparation for strenuous gardening work.

This area is enclosed by pleached trees that screen out an unsightly neighbouring building and afford privacy. In this formation, the trees take up less space and light than if they were allowed to grow naturally.

Four ornamental trees set in box-edged beds help to create a restful courtyard space. This area is ideal for eating, relaxing, or performing an outdoor exercise routine.

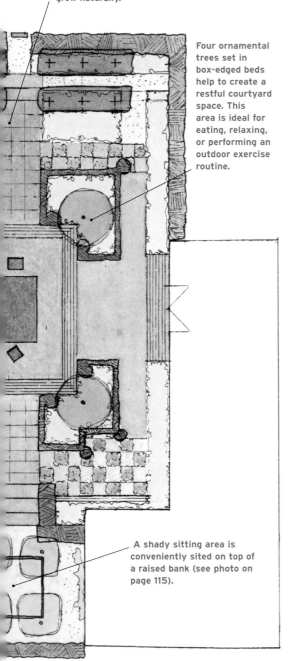

A shady sitting area is conveniently sited on top of a raised bank (see photo on page 115).

A SAMPLE MASTER PLAN

Useable spaces feature heavily in this garden plan, designed for a family with three energetic children. A treehouse, informal pool with boardwalk, trampoline, large lawn, and winding path encourage physical activity, while an eating area and an unusual flying-saucer-shaped swing (see page 65) invite relaxation, and a fruit orchard and vegetable garden give generous scope for growing healthy food. Although there is a lot going on in this garden, the maintenance that it requires is not overwhelming.

DRAWING A MASTER PLAN

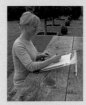

Even the drawing of a master plan for your garden can be done in a way that reduces the risk of strain. As anyone who spends long periods in front of a computer or writing at a desk will know, a prolonged period in this position often leads to pain in the back and the neck.

The equipment you choose will affect your posture. Try to select a drawing board that can be positioned at any angle, so that you are not compelled to stoop over it. An even better posture can be achieved using a chair 6–8 in. (15–20 cm) higher than usual. Additionally, try arranging your seat and desktop so that they slope towards one another; this angle opens up your hip joint and encourages your lumbar curve (lower back) to maintain its healthy neutral position. Other ergonomic options include a forward-tilting seat that lets your hips stay slightly higher than your knees, a seat wedge, and a desk slope. A bar or footstool on which to place your feet will also prevent your legs from being suspended in midair. All of this equipment serves to prevent slumping, helping you to avoid back and neck pain and breathe more thoroughly.

Try not to become so absorbed in your work that you lose track of time and end up staying in the sitting position for too long; as with sustained activity in the garden, you should get up, take a break, and walk around regularly to avoid strain. Forty minutes is the maximum time period you should spend working on your master plan before taking a break.

If you do not have a drawing board, then a piece of medium-density fibreboard (MDF) with your sheet of paper clipped onto it will also work. If you use a computer to list problems that you wish to camouflage or features that you want to add or enhance, raise the screen on some books to bring it to eye level, reducing the need to stoop. The computer should always be directly in front of you so that you do not need to twist at an angle to see it, and the keyboard and mouse should be straight in front of you rather than set off to the side.

Walkways

Paths lead you around the garden, connecting up the various spaces so that the whole garden interrelates. At the start of a gardening session, a saunter around your garden's path network will let you check up on the wellbeing of your plants, admire what is in flower, and assess what needs to be deadheaded, weeded, or pruned. If you move at a brisk pace, this can serve as your pre-gardening warmup or part of your aerobic routine. Because you will probably see and use your paths every day, it is worth taking time to determine what kind of paths you want, how you want them to look, and which functions you want each of your paths to serve.

You may use some routes several times a day—for instance, the route down to the greenhouse, or up to the chicken coop if you have one—while other routes are used less frequently but serve more aesthetic purposes by leading the eye on to an attractive gate, seat, or arbour. The route leading to the compost heap should be a fairly direct one, and it should be wide enough for a heavily laden barrow and free of steps and awkward obstacles. Additionally, you may want to add subsidiary paths which are only a brick's length wide—just wide enough to afford access to the back of border for maintenance use only.

RIGHT: A checkerboard effect is created by combining paving with squares of *Thymus serpyllum* 'Minimalist'.

BELOW: Indian stone setts measuring 4 × 4 in. (10 × 10 cm) line this path. They are especially useful for making smaller areas appear larger.

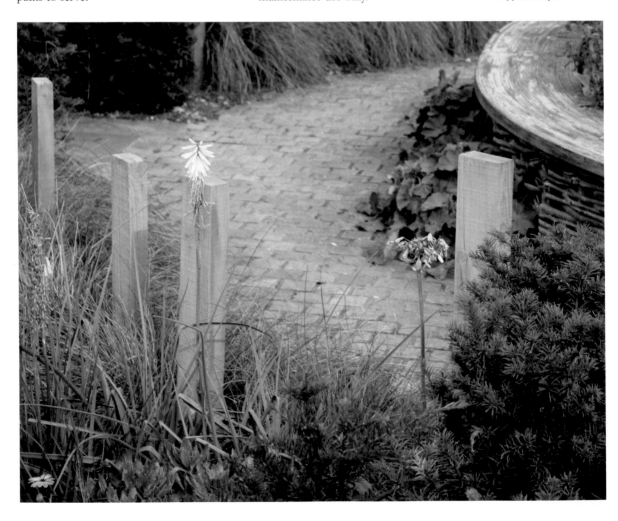

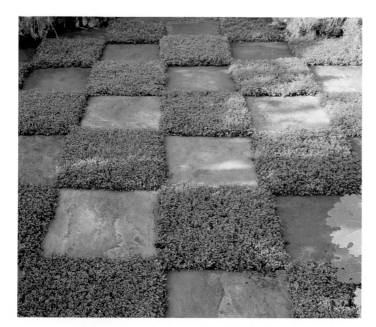

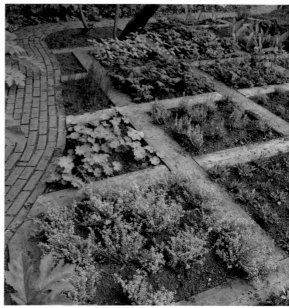

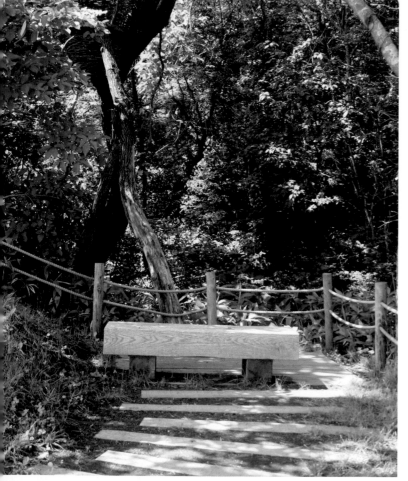

LEFT: Sunken sleepers are laid informally, leading to an exercise bench that looks down onto a river. A woven treetop 'nest' provides an exhilarating lookout point.

ABOVE: Miniature paths of sunken sleepers are perfect for dividing up these small beds of vegetables and herbs.

Paths may be wide, overstated, heavily structured, and hard, or they may be low-key affairs with just a narrow width of mown grass between borders or areas of flowering meadow. When it comes to materials for pathways, many options are available. A checkerboard of paving slabs in grass, gravel, crushed cockle shells, crushed glass, sand, cocoa shells or bark would all work well. Alternatively, sunken sleepers or slabs arranged in an interesting pattern and laid flush with the lawn add distinction to the pathways that lead around the garden.

Not many people have a network of paths that is long enough to jog around, but it may be worth incorporating a few logs, steps, seats, and beams in a logical sequence. These will be ideal for exercising, stretching, and working out various parts of your body in the fresh air, whenever you have a spare moment. You may even want to create your own trim trail (see Chapter 2). If your garden is small, a network of miniature paths with a trim trail nearby can be used for circuit training.

Walkways

When you use certain parts of the garden frequently, it does not take long before grass wears thin and turns to mud. One approach is to wait and see which routes become worn, and then step in to resolve the problem by installing a hard surface. Designing in subtle twists and bends can create a naturalistic feel and you can open up other areas more as you define a slightly less direct route.

Walkways bring out the potential of your garden. You may have a lovely orchard, a soothing wildlife pool, or a stunning rose garden, but it is the paths that link them up that will encourage these spaces to be used as much as possible. Paths can be designed to be highly attractive elements in themselves, whether they are narrow and shady, curving and informal, or wide, welcoming and sunny. Decide what personality and style would suit that area and develop the path so that it not only ties the formal bones of the garden together and makes it function, but also helps the various areas of your garden to come into their own and brings about a series of exciting experiences as you wander, jog, or garden your way around your space.

Deep lavender-filled beds flank this wide pathway while metal-archways provide a strong vertical element.

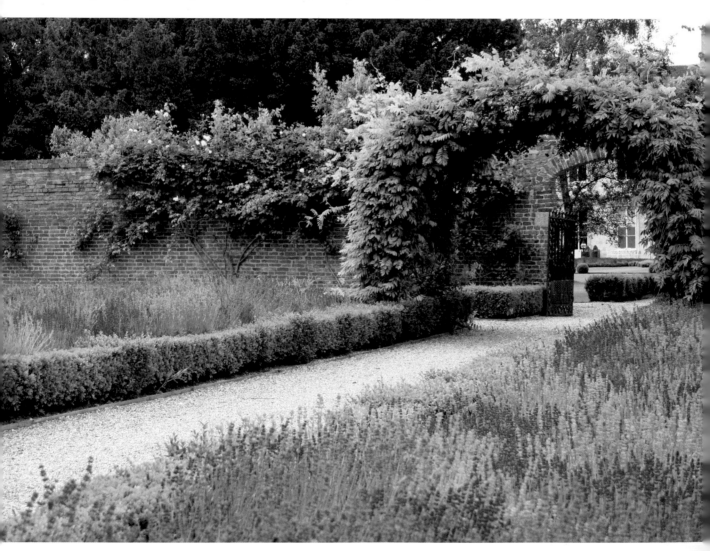

Levels

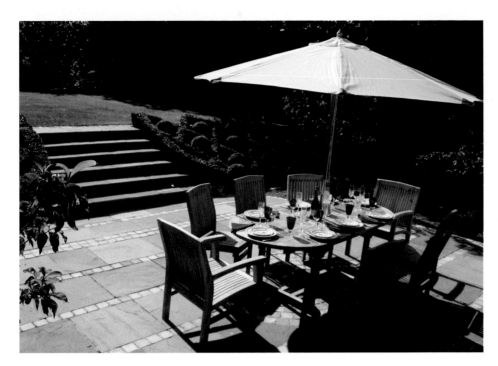

Slopes, steps, and high viewing points add interest to your space and make you feel exhilarated, but this is only part of their appeal. Your garden's varying levels (and the steps and slopes you use to negotiate them) can also help to boost your fitness levels; running up steps and slopes can burn a serious quantity of calories if done regularly and vigorously.

Yet although using the levels in your garden as exercise spaces can be great for your body, it is important not to do too much, too suddenly. Like any aerobic exercise, it makes sense to carry out this type of exercise gently (working up gradually to longer sequences), and often; doing it a few times a week for ten minutes at a time will make more sense than overexerting yourself in one marathon exercise session over the weekend.

It is important to do this on a regular basis to maintain strength and range of movement in your thigh muscles, as when you stop going up and down steps your joints tend to stiffen up and these muscles can become weak.

Even if you are not inclined to use the levels in your garden to exercise, you can still maximize them visually. High planting on top of a bank or retaining wall will emphasize its stature, whereas planting at its base will lessen its perceived height. You can use the levels in your garden to divide an otherwise sprawling or expansive space up into interesting areas.

ACCENTUATING SLOPES

When you first glance at a space, you do not always notice its slight variations in level. Some lawns simply register as annoyingly not-quite-flat, rather restless spaces where ball games are awkward; in cases such as these, there may be quite a difference in levels even if it is barely perceptible. It is worth checking the levels in your garden (perhaps by hiring a laser level) to see whether there is scope for manipulating them.

By accentuating the differences in level that already exist, you can make the spaces in your garden more suitable for relaxation as well as exercise.

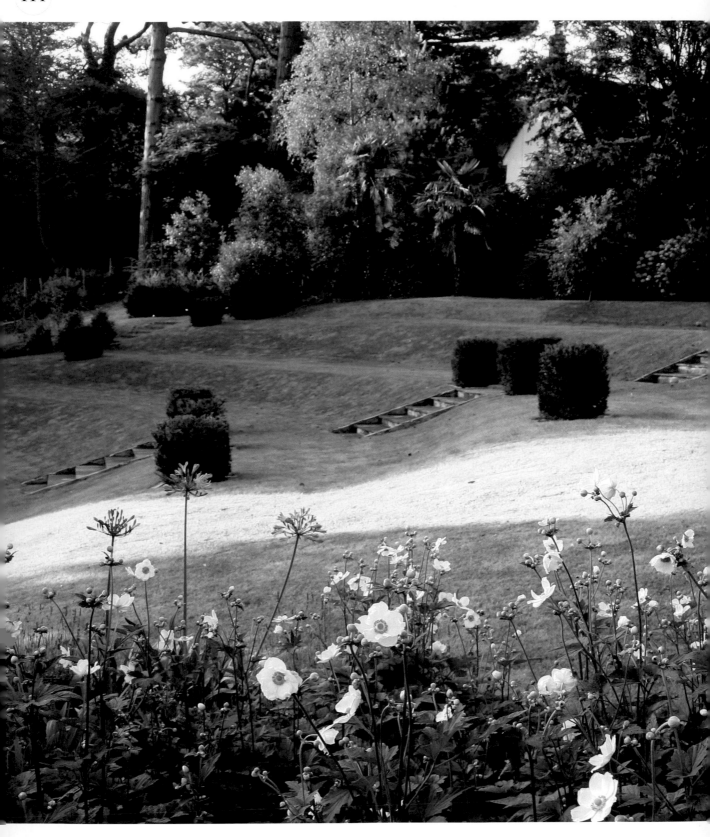

The process of accentuating levels may involve cutting into a subtle slope to create a more useable flat space with a bank or wall to take up the slope. This adds to the drama of the space and often creates viable exercise areas. You can greatly increase the privacy of spaces, too, by reducing the level where privacy is required and using the material gained from that reduction to create higher levels around the perimeter. Planting tall screen plants on top of the higher levels creates a sense of seclusion.

On sites exposed to winds and gales, you can instantly form sheltered areas by sinking seating areas, especially when you add planting on the newly created higher and more exposed areas to help filter out the wind. Steps, banks, and raised platforms add that intriguing touch of elevation, and of course they are useful for adding challenge and variety to your 'outdoor gym'.

STEPS

In addition to being useful as informal spots for sitting, steps offer options for exercise that target the muscles in your calves and thighs. Walking up and down stairs at a slow to moderate pace is a great way to warm up, and quickening your gait makes for a calorie-burning aerobic workout. A single step is a great place for practising step-ups, as long as the step is not so high that your knee has to bend at an angle greater than 90° in order to step onto it.

Making the steps wide and spacious creates a generous, expansive, and leisurely feel. To reduce maintenance, placing a generous mowing edge around all parts of the step that abut grass (sides, top, and bottom) will help you to avoid all of that tedious edging work that would cause you to stoop over uncomfortably.

Steps can also be made to look soft, if you opt for grass treads (treads being the part of the step you put your feet on) and timber risers (that is, the vertical parts of the stairs)—just make sure that the treads are at least as wide as your mower. By adding dwarf hedging, you can mask the timber to make the stairs appear completely green.

Alternatively, you can incorporate low hedging as a replacement for side walls by 'sitting' the steps into the bank.

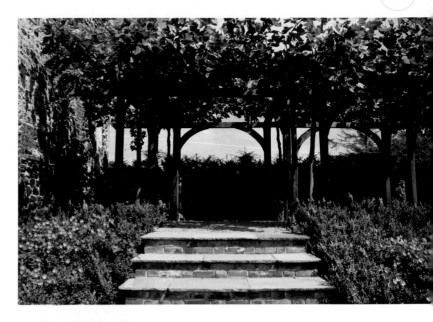

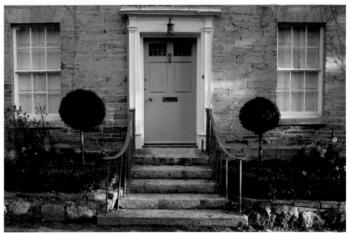

Safety on the Steps

Although steep, narrow steps add a feeling of exhilaration, safety can be an issue, especially in wet or icy weather—and these types of steps are particularly inadvisable when they are to be used by small children, or by those who are not especially nimble on their feet. Avoiding slippery materials such as sleepers and large units of stone slabs, especially in shady situations where algae and moss colonize, is a must. For these areas, a smaller unit paving like granite setts or bricks with regular joints between the units allows the foot to grip.

Handrails may also be included for extra safety. These are usually placed about 3 ft. (90 cm) above the steps. If you do not

LEFT: These 25° banks can be mown with a rotary mower. A stone slab mowing margin gives the steps a clean, crisp look.

TOP: This elevated shady sitting area is made of chunky green oak posts and beams, punctuated by tabletop-trained plane trees to 'green up' the structure.

ABOVE: This delicate metal handrail contrasts nicely with the bold granite steps.

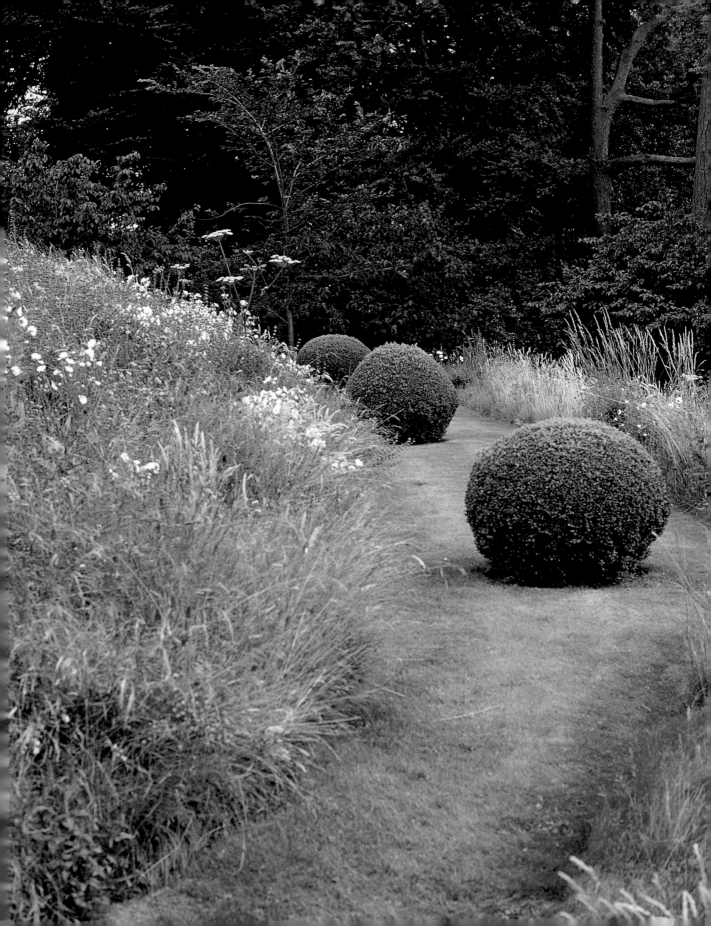

have a side wall, an elegant solution is a single simple rail. If the handrails can be incorporated into a side wall, they are generally less intrusive. For steps that you are planning to use on a regular basis, it is best to keep riser heights low. Heights of more than 7 in. (30 cm) can cause problems and are best avoided.

Options for Making Banks

Reworking your outdoor space to accentuate differences in level often requires that you build banks or retaining walls. Retaining walls are not always the best choice, as they can be harsh-looking and expensive to install. Banks, on the other hand, are inexpensive. Whether they are mown or planted, it is important that they be designed carefully to prevent any problematic maintenance issues from emerging.

Turf banks are a simple and low-key option. Once you have obtained your turves, you will need to kill off the grass by either using glyphosate or leaving the grass under black polythene for approximately one month. The next step is to construct a wall using the upside-down pieces of turf, laying them one on top of the other like bricks, with staggered joints. The wall could be up to about 1 ft. (30 cm) wide, but not much higher. The bank should slope back slightly, making it more stable. You can then plant ferns, ivy, or *Vinca minor* into the cracks, soaking them well initially and then watering them until they take root in the mass. Eventually, these plants will colonize the slope and help to stabilize it. You can stud the banks with gnarled roots and sow primroses on them if desired.

Another 'soft' option is to grow a battered and slightly sloping woven willow wall. You can do this by pushing vertical rods into the ground at roughly 6 in. (15 cm) centres. Then, weave horizontal rods through them, pushing the base ends back into the soil so that they take root. The bank should be set at a slight slope to give it greater stability. The growing willow will need to be cut back up to five times each year; when you do so, you can strengthen the framework by weaving in new shoots. In time, the woven parts all fuse together, grafting themselves to one another so that a solid framework emerges.

Planted banks are a popular option, and because no mowing is necessary they allow you to achieve a steeper angle (even as steep as 45°). If you do not want to draw attention to the bank, you can plant a hedge at its base. The planting that colonizes the soil on the bank will be hidden behind the hedge and therefore hardly visible, so a monoculture of a bland, weed-suppressing plant such as ivy (*Hedera helix*) or a good, low strain of comfrey (*Symphytum* 'Hidcote Blue') will work well—they are easy to establish and maintain. Weeding steep banks can be tricky, so to avoid aggravation you should ensure that the soil is as weed-free as possible at the outset.

Grass Slopes

Mown slopes can look superb, especially when they are formed into a series of regular and uniform banks that punctuate a number of horizontal platforms with broad brush strokes. To save yourself frustration during the maintenance process, it is important to design the slopes so they are not too steep for your mower to manoeuvre. The slope should be no steeper than 25° if you use a petrol rotary mower (whether it the kind that you ride or walk behind), 20° for a cylinder (reel) mower (which is limited by the lubrication of its engine), or 45° for a hover mower. With a strimmer (weed-whacker), on the other hand, you can tackle a slope at any angle, as long as you are able to stand on it. Mowing these slopes is more aerobic than mowing level lawns.

Make sure that the design is slick. For instance, you really do not want grass banks to be butting against vertical walls to steps, leaving you with edges that need cutting with shears, so try to put in a mowing edge if possible.

If you want a particularly eye-catching bank, you can make it into a wildflower meadow, which will look stunning when the flowers are shown off at an angle. If you are creating the bank from scratch, then you should take the opportunity to leave poorer subsoil on the bank as this will encourage wildflower growth while discouraging the growth of vigorous grass. (For more information on maintaining the balance between weeds and more desirable plants in wildflower meadows, turn to the end of this chapter.)

LEFT: **Wildflowers look good and often do very well on a bank. Here the closely mown grass and clipped box balls show off the lax nature of the long grass.**

Paving and Gravel

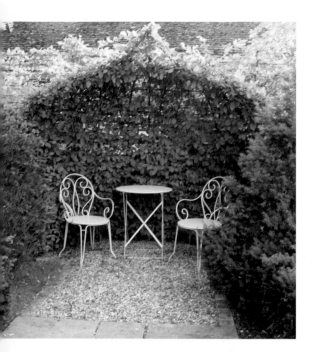

In addition to serving as welcoming spaces for eating, drinking, and entertaining, hard surfaces such as paving and gravel are ideal for quick workouts when the grass is unuseable. They can lend the garden an air of being an 'outdoor gym', allowing quick bursts of aerobic activity such as step-ups, running on the spot and many other exercises to be shoehorned into odd moments during your daily routine.

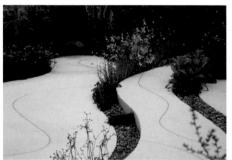

FAR LEFT: This gravel path leads to a hornbeam arbour. The trees are trained over a lightweight metal framework.

LEFT: In this garden designed by Sarah Eberle, a large area of concrete paving is effectively broken up by gravel and planting. The paving's dynamic, sinuous shape softens its impact and metal bands emphasize its shapely curves.

BELOW: This 2-ft. (60-cm) stone ball looks attractive and is convenient for stretching.

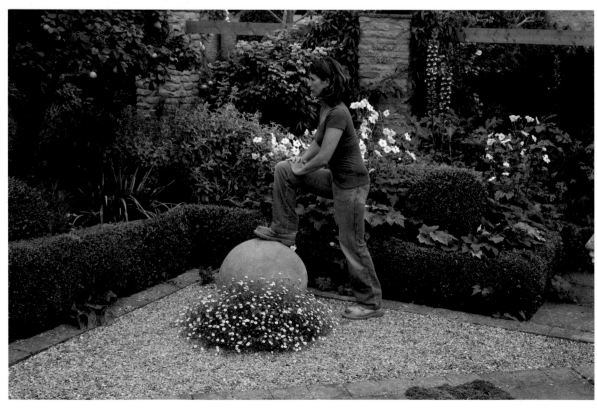

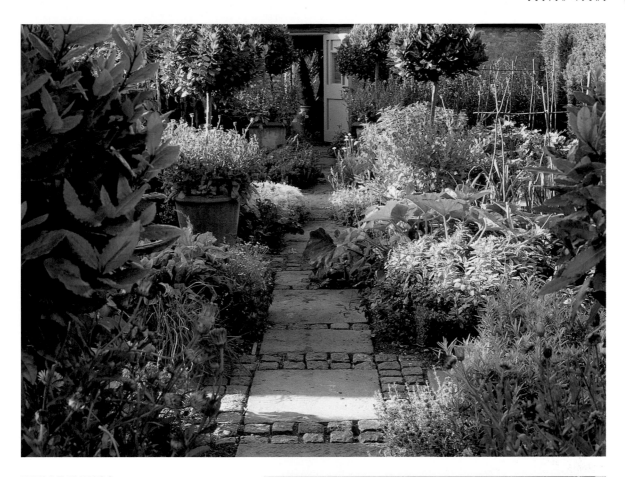

WHY PAVING?

In addition to being eminently useable, generously proportioned and well-designed paved areas bring a strong sense of structure to the garden. Their appeal stays constant in all weather and throughout the changing seasons.

Gardeners who are highly pressed for time are often particularly fond of hard surfaces because they are virtually maintenance-free once installed. Paved areas tend to wear well, retaining an excellent finish for many, many years, largely regardless of how they are maintained.

The main disadvantage of paving is its high initial cost: expensive paving may well cost ten times the amount of a basic planted border. However, after paving is installed its maintenance costs are basically nonexistent—and by mixing a small amount of the more pricey paving with larger areas of less expensive paving (such as gravel) you can make a paved area considerably more affordable.

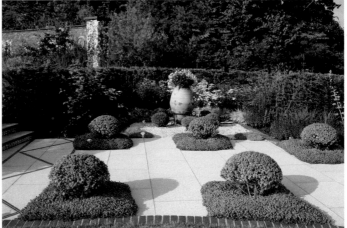

TOP: **This path measures 2 ft. (60 cm) across—just wide enough for a wheelbarrow. A stone-and-granite-sett mix is a good alternative to grass paths, which are prone to becoming muddy and can cause extra work when the grass invades nearby planting beds.**

ABOVE: **Paving slabs are broken up by box balls surrounded by thyme, and purple tiles placed on end form a zigzag pattern between slabs.**

Paving and Gravel

GRAVEL

Gravel is usually inexpensive and looks equally fantastic in front of a castle or a cottage. It makes for a great 'outdoor gym' surface, and when you carry out aerobic exercise on it, gravel can be slightly more sympathetic to your joints. Some people are wary of gravel, though, because of its annoying tendency to be picked up on shoes and then dragged into buildings, and if it is laid too deeply it can wreck high-heeled shoes.

However, this can be avoided if you design the spaces that lead into doorways with solid paving and make sure that the top-wearing course is of minimal thickness. This top-wearing course should be laid onto a compacted, blinded hardcore base.

GRAVEL AND PAVING

Alternatively, you may opt for bound gravel, which does not attach itself to shoes. Bound gravel surfaces are fixed and stable enough for wheelchairs, tricycles, and even high heels.

Some are bound with a clear resin-type material, but these tend to be very expensive and almost too perfect-looking. Others contain fine clay articles and are watered well on laying, causing the clay to rise to the surface, and when they are subsequently rolled they bind the surface. This type of gravel is produced by only a few quarries nowadays (see Appendix).

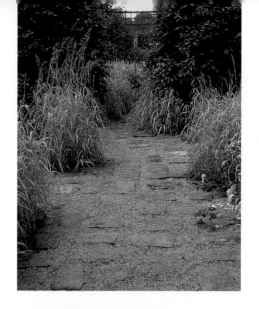

Here gravel is broken up by chunky granite setts, which create a striking effect when juxtaposed with tall grasses.

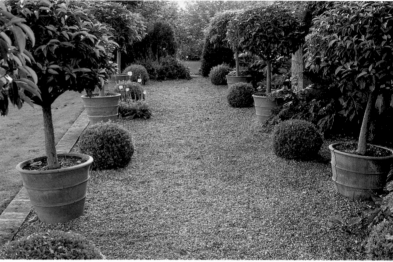

ABOVE: Bricks form a clean edge to this gravel path which is lined with clipped laurels in bottomless terracotta pots.

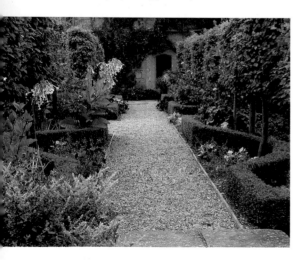

LEFT: Here the gravel is edged by timber and the curvy line of the box makes the path seem wider.

GRAVEL FOR SAFETY

Gravel can also function as a safety surface underneath swings, climbing frames, and treehouses. While the gravel used for paving typically has angular particles so that these tiny pieces can be bound together, the gravel used for safety surfaces has rounded particles with cushioning air spaces between them, forming a shock-absorbent surface.

When you are laying gravel as a safety surface, you will need a greater depth of the wearing surface (1 ft. [30 cm]), and the rounded particles should measure ⅛–½ in. (3–13 mm) in diameter. Unfortunately, such deep gravel would wreak havoc on high heels, and would require regular raking to maintain its neat appearance. However, it makes an excellent surface for an aerobic workout.

Lawns and Their Maintenance

The grassed areas of a garden will strongly define its overall character. Different maintenance treatments give rise to very different styles, from a laid-back flowery meadow to rigid, emerald stripes. Before you commit yourself to several hours a week behind or on a mower, think carefully about the effect you want to achieve.

Some countries are historically more fastidious about maintaining their lawns than others. In England and the United States, having a pristine, green, striped lawn resembling a pool (snooker) table used to symbolize that all was exactly as it should be. Recently, though, gardeners' eyes have opened up radically to looser, lower-maintenance options for grassy areas.

Not only can these provide a more appealing backcloth to a garden, but they require fewer expensive pieces of equipment and less chemical treatment. Allowing grass to grow longer will also encourage wildlife to visit the garden. One eminent British gardener, the late Christopher Lloyd, was responsible for converting many traditionalists when he transformed his billiard-table lawns into wildflower meadows. The only rule of thumb, then, is to allow yourself the freedom to experiment and indulge in the approach you find most appropriate to the amount of space you have available (and the amount of time that you want to spend maintaining it).

Taking small measures can improve your lawn's appearance greatly; for instance, if your garden is quite compact and the grassy area is limited, you can make the lawn look special by raising the soil by about 4 in. (10 cm) and putting an attractive edge around it to retain it. This edge may be made from various materials such as steel, a brick turned on its side, or a chunky piece of green oak timber. Combining this with a path will prevent the grassy area from turning into a muddy patch as it is continually traipsed over.

If you have a large garden and are pressed for time, you can allow certain areas to grow marginally longer while others are meticulously groomed, which evokes a

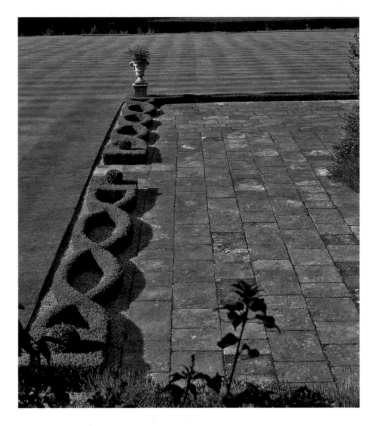

unique atmosphere and reduces cutting time significantly. With this approach you need to use a mulching mower (where you leave the mini, shredded cuttings on) or a rotary mower that is capable of collecting grass at a longer length of about 4 in (10 cm), to attain a good contrast with shorter, more useable grass.

Wildflower meadows are a further, and even more relaxed, option; although they are certainly not easy (they are difficult to get 'right' initially), they are relaxing to live with and fabulous for attracting wildlife. Ecolawns are yet another relatively low-maintenance option, demanding less work than traditional lawns while still being highly useable. These three lower-maintenance grassy options are explored further at the end of this chapter, and the following section explains how to carry out the various lawn maintenance procedures in a safe and healthy way.

This high-maintenance lawn has been mown with a cylinder (reel) mower and demands regular feeding, scarifying, and applications of herbicides and moss killers to keep it looking weed-free and attractive.

Lawns and Their Maintenance

LAWN MAINTENANCE

Lawn mowing and the collection of leaves and cuttings are central to lawn care. Using a strimmer (weed-whacker) allows you to tackle grass and weeds in tight spaces that most mowers cannot reach, while edging can really define a grassy area, making it look polished and enticing. Raking—a task that is often vigorous, yet also very satisfying—keeps the lawn tidy.

Starting and Pushing a Power Mower

Mowing the lawn is an excellent way to burn calories, but starting a power mower is a somewhat tricky manoeuvre in that it can easily strain your lower back and neck. Following this advice will help you to benefit from the mowing 'workout' without damaging your body.

• **Avoid gripping the handles too hard as this stresses your forearms.**

• **While you are pushing the mower, the impetus and strength should come from your stomach rather than your back, as much as possible. This is where a strong, engaged core comes in handy; keeping your abdominal muscles pulled up and in will help to protect your back.**

• **Gardeners have a tendency to lean on the handles when tired. Avoid doing this as it can lead to strain in your neck, shoulders, and lower back. Instead, take a break whenever you find yourself beginning to grow weary.**

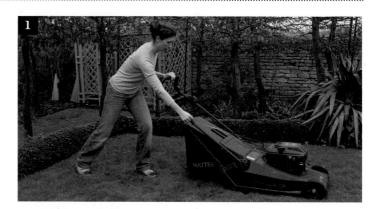

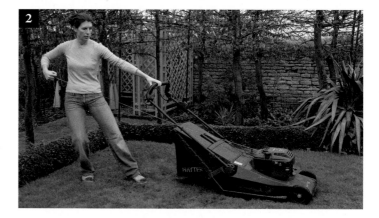

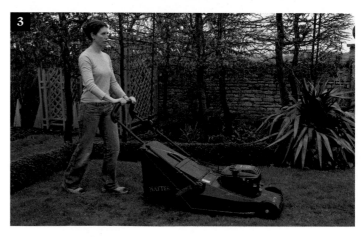

1 Begin with your back in neutral and your shoulder blades down and in. Stand with your legs in a wide stance so that you have a good base of support; one leg should be positioned behind the other. Then, reach for the cord of the power mower.

2 Drawing your lower stomach muscles up and in, rotate through your thorax and use your oblique abdominal muscles as you pull the starter cord towards you, shifting your weight onto your back leg.

3 As you push the mower your shoulder blades should be set down towards the centre of your upper back, while your lower abdominal muscles should be lifted up and in, supporting your lower back. This way your abdominal muscles and shoulder blades, rather than your lower back and neck, drive the movement.

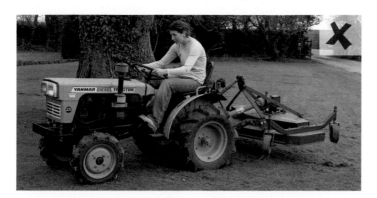

Using a Ride-on (Riding) Mower

When sitting on a ride-on (riding) mower your spine should be in neutral. Your shoulder blades should be back, down, and in, which again takes the stress off your neck. If you get tired, do not slouch or slump. Instead, take a break: get off the mower and stand tall. Walk around for a few minutes, maintaining an upright posture. You might even stretch up towards the sky with your hands.

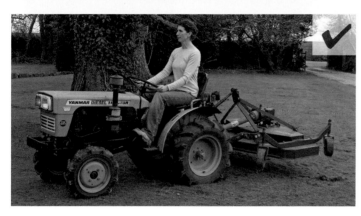

ABOVE LEFT: **In this position, you risk straining your back and your neck.**

LEFT: **Make sure your spine is in neutral, and that your shoulders are back.**

Strimming (Weed-Whacking)

A long-handled strimmer (weed-whacker) will help protect you from the need to bend over, which can strain your back and neck. Try to maintain an upright posture and keep your lower back in its neutral position. The key to maintaining a neutral spine is the height of the strimmer, which should be just below your waist so that your arms can grasp the handle while slightly bent.

When using a strimmer, a visor and earmuffs are crucial, and a face mask and gloves should also be worn. Cordless strimmers are easier to use because there is no cable to avoid, but are only useful on small areas. If your strimmer has a cable, you should also wear a cable safe, which is a safety harness that helps to guard against accidents that could be caused by trailing electric cables.

Often gardeners keep their feet rooted to the ground while swinging their strimmers from side to side, twisting their backs in the process. This technique should be avoided as the rotation places too much stress on your lower back. Instead, your feet should be continuously moving back and forth as you change direction, enabling your spine to remain straight. Lift your lower abdominal muscles up and in, so that these muscles receive a gentle workout. (The same advice applies when using a hover mower.)

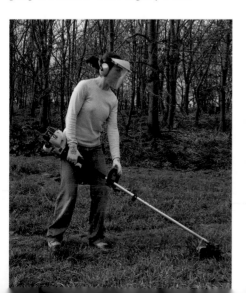

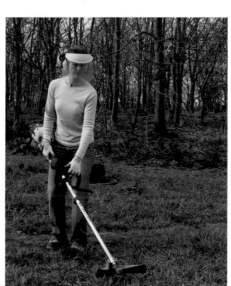

Edging

Edges of lawns abutting soil can easily become messy if grass creeps into the adjacent soil or evades the mower's blades where the lawn abuts a wall, steps, building, fencepost, or tree. One way to deal with this is to carefully manicure these edges by hand, but this can be high-maintenance and fiddly, as well as potentially damaging to your back and neck as it often involves crouching over the ground for substantial periods of time. To avoid having to do this, you may wish to add a mowing margin.

In the absence of a mowing margin, edging will need to be carried out approximately every other time you mow your lawn (although some would advise doing it each time you mow). Long-handled edging shears, or any shears with adjustable handles), are good tools for keeping the area crisp.

An edger in a half-moon shape or a sharp spade can be used to re-cut a raggedy lawn edge, perhaps once a year. There are also mechanical tools for cutting the edge of the grass; cordless shears, which you need to bend or kneel to use, are very lightweight, efficient, and easy to manoeuvre. Nylon line trimmers are also useful—the easiest ones to use come with clip-on wheels that maintain a set height above the ground, or a head that rotates to cut vertically.

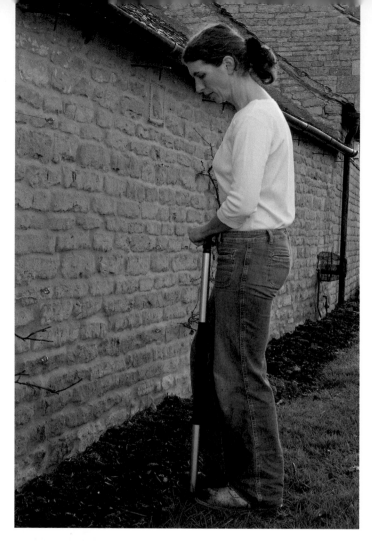

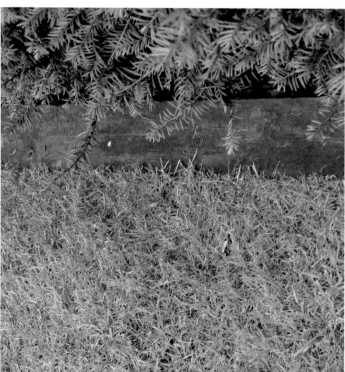

LEFT: This substantial mowing edge was created by using a railway sleeper set about 0.2 in. (5 mm) below the surface of the turf. This allows you to run the edge of the mower along the edge of the sleeper, eliminating the need for time-consuming (and potentially back-breaking) edging work with shears.

ABOVE: As you push down on the edger with one foot, keep your shoulder blades down and in to diminish any strain on your neck.

Raking

Raking may be necessary for removing leaves or cuttings from a lawn, or to freshen up gravel—and if it is performed with good technique it is great exercise. It uses the muscles of the entire upper body including your shoulders, the pectorals across your chest, and your abdominal and back muscles. It is important to keep the rake in easy reach by keeping the action close to your body. Do not overstretch.

Bending down to pick up the leaves will also work your legs and bottom, and discourage you from stooping. Try to alternate sides for a more balanced workout. This is difficult and requires considerable coordination!

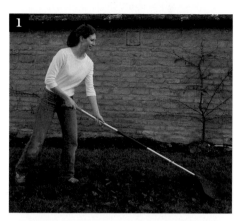

1 Start in an upright position with your feet hip-width apart and hands shoulder-width apart, one in front of the other. Move with the rake so that it is rather like doing a lunge, with one leg coming forward as you shift weight onto it. Your back remains in its neutral position.

2 Lift the rake and place it over the leaves in preparation for pulling them back towards you.

3 As you pull the rake towards your body, draw momentum by shifting weight from your front leg onto your back foot and lifting your lower abdominals inward to protect your lower back.

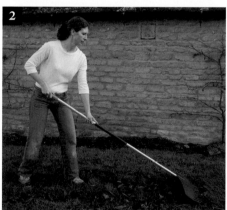

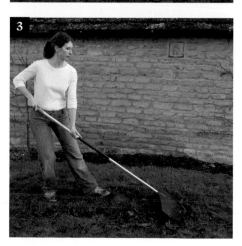

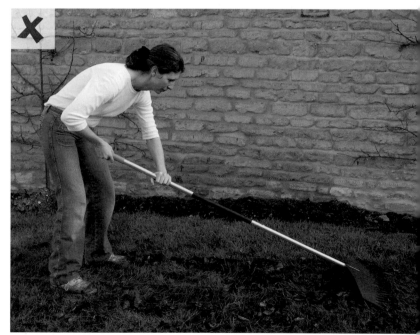

ABOVE: **If you bend over like this, you place unnecessary strain on your back, neck, and shoulders.**

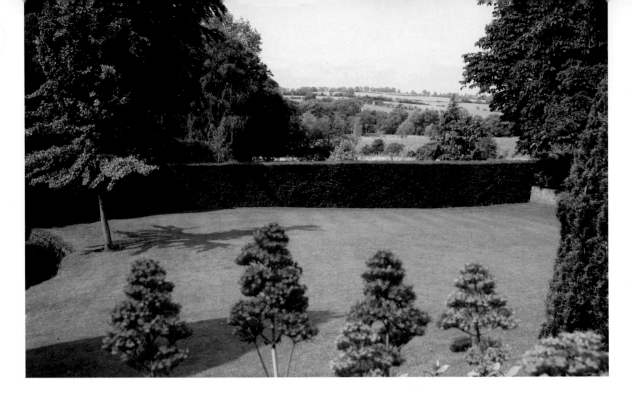

YOUR GRASSY GYM

Running on the lawn is an excellent way to exercise. Grass is more forgiving on the knee joints, and feeling it underneath our toes makes us feel really rooted to the earth. Spending a few minutes doing deep breathing tends to be significantly more relaxing when performed on a lawn as opposed to a hard surface, and because grass is so soft it is ideal for lying on when you carry out Pilates body-balancing work.

Although many gardens are not spacious enough for tennis courts or swimming pools, it is often possible to improvise. For instance, relatively inexpensive, inflatable swimming pools can be put up on any convenient paved area during the summer. For limited periods where it will be well-used, this option is worth having (even if it is a bit of eyesore).

Setting up nets for tennis, badminton, or cricket, or even a ping-pong table helps to bring out the potential of your grassy space, and of course a swingset or jungle gym set on a mown, grassy surface will encourage children to exercise in the fresh air.

Protecting Your Lawn and Plants

Mown lawns are natural magnets for energetic, ball-mad boys and girls, which is wonderful as children draw huge benefit from being out in the fresh air. Yet if your lawn is highly manicured and surrounded by elaborate planting, you may feel an element of conflict between the urge to encourage active play and the desire to protect the grass and surrounding area.

To avoid this kind of stress, it helps to design the area around your lawn in a way that minimizes the risk of damage. For the area bordering the lawn, choose less delicate plants, including lower-level herbaceous plants such as geraniums, daylilies, and catmint, as well as tougher shrubs like germander, hollies, and shrub roses. Planting beds with low hedging helps, too: not only does it define the lawn's edge, but it also helps to screen the vulnerable plants. In confined gardens, you may want to limit ball games to the dormant season when the herbaceous plants are safely underground. Adding alternative play elements (for instance, a sunken trampoline) away from the lawn is a clever tactic, as it takes some of the pressure off of the grass.

To keep the grass in good condition, the soil should be well-draining—and make sure the turf is a hard-wearing one by opting for a dwarf rye grass mix. As the lawn is often a place where everyone congregates, informal seating areas such as generous steps, enticing grass banks or a large circular seat around a fabulous specimen tree will all enhance the space.

This clean, green central area is an inviting space for exercise. It acts as a visual 'breathing space' within a complex garden.

LOWER-MAINTENANCE GRASSY SPACES

Keeping lawns in shape has traditionally involved not only mowing but also a myriad of other maintenance tasks, from removing unwanted weeds, to scarifying the area to remove a thatch buildup, to applying moss killers and fertilizers and even removing coarser grasses.

However, taking a high-maintenance approach to lawn care is certainly not a must and in recent years it has even become unfashionable due to the amount of chemicals and the amount of upkeep that these strategies require. Reducing the areas that need to be cut frequently will save time, energy, and stress, and cutting down on mowing also helps to decrease your carbon footprint.

When grasses are allowed to grow more freely, uniquely enjoyable spaces can emerge. These may be flowering meadows (cut once or twice a year), longer grass (cut every three weeks or so in the growing season), or ecolawns (cut frequently but omitting traditional maintenance regimes). You can play around with the balance of differently maintained grassy areas to discover what works best for you.

Wildflower Meadows

A wildflower meadow—consisting of a low-maintenance stretch of longer grass dotted with wildflowers and herbs—can become a beacon to wildlife. These meadows are fun to develop, and they are very satisfying once you achieve a desirable balance between weeds and flowers.

The success or failure of flowering meadows depends on the preparation you undertake. Ideally, grass, flowers, and herbs should be established on less fertile soil where the population of pernicious weed seeds—those highly invasive, less-than-attractive plants like nettles, docks, creeping thistles, and Japanese knotweed—is minimal. You should remove these and all other weeds at the outset, perhaps during a fallow period where you allow the weeds to germinate and then kill them off before they set seed.

To encourage the wildflower seeds to establish, sow a low density of grass seed. Many gardeners have difficulty with wildflower seed sown directly; to avoid

frustration you may prefer to plant in plugs of wildflowers, which may be homegrown or bought from a garden centre.

To save even more time and cut down on preparation work, you can create an instant flowering meadow by using areas of ready-growing wildflower and grass swards that come on a thin felt mixture that quickly degrades after establishment. Although this is expensive, it has the bonus of suppressing all of the existing weed seeds.

These areas may become untidy once the amazing flower show is over and you have to leave the unruly-looking mass to set seed for next year before you cut it. The task of cutting is usually undertaken with a nylon cord trimmer. However, the cutting can be made easier if you have a trimmer mower, which is pushed on two wheels. This is a tough machine that will not be damaged by odd bricks and other unexpected surprises that you may stumble over during these very infrequent cutting sessions.

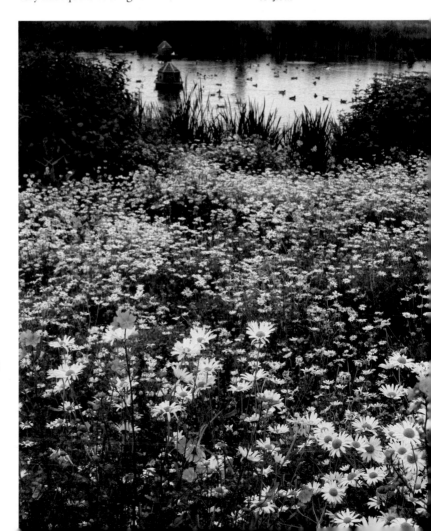

These perennial ox-eye (or 'moon') daisies look spectacular en masse and are believed to have a wide range of medicinal uses. At dusk or in moonlight the daisies really seem to glow.

To achieve a satisfying mixture of grass, flowers, and herbs, as opposed to an explosion of coarser weeds like dandelions, you may need to carry out selective weeding initially. If your lawn is near a large population of less desirable weeds (often found in fields and woodland), then they may continue to creep in.

This issue can be combatted by using a knapsack- or hand-held sprayer and simply spot-treating the offenders. A daisy grubber with a forked blade for reaching under taproots is an organic alternative.

Many coarse weeds will slide out easily if you tackle them after heavy rain—just be sure to wear gauntlets to protect your arms. By keeping the lawn's fertility level low, weeding selectively, and removing the cuttings after the annual cut, you can slowly shift the balance in favour of the wildflowers. Annual wildflowers such as

poppies will dominate in the first year, after which they will die out unless you disturb the soil in places. Perennial wildflowers rarely bloom from seed in their first year, but they can slowly gather momentum from their second year onwards. Yellow rattle (*Rhinanthus minor*) is an attractive annual that is semi-parasitic of grasses; try sowing it in autumn to curb the grass growth, which in turn will allow the wildflowers to flourish.

Every year, these low-maintenance spaces will be different; they are often one of the most dynamic parts of a garden. They afford huge scope to be creative, as you can experiment by planting all manner of bulbs and natural-looking plants in them.

The fabulous thing about these wilder spaces is you can do as much or little as you like. If the grassy areas are relatively small, you can gently manicure them so they retain their relaxed, bohemian character without becoming too wild and woolly. In the early years it may be necessary to hand weed out more pernicious weeds such as nettles and creeping thistles.

For best results, carry out this weeding when the weeds are young, and preferably after rainfall. If the grassy edges flop over the mown paths too much for your liking, you can simply trim them back now and then with a pair of shears.

Longer Grass

If a wildflower meadow is a bit too wayward for your tastes, another option is to cut the grass to a length of about 4 in. (10 cm), cutting every two or three weeks during the growing season. This treatment gives rise to a informal grassy areas that are more manageable than meadows, yet require significantly less cutting than lawns do.

Because more frequent cutting of grass stimulates growth, you will find that this slightly longer grass grows more sedately. You can add an element of artistry by adding interesting and useful closely mown paths to contrast with the longer grass. There should be no need to fertilize this grass, nor should you need to roll it or scarify it. Quite a few wildflowers such as the pencilled crane's bill (*Geranium versicolor*) may also thrive under this regime, adding to the tapestry effect. In the wild many of these herbaceous plants survive being grazed, so a regular light chop will

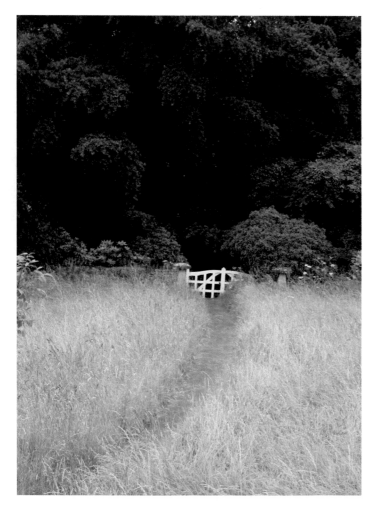

A mown path winds through the long grass in this low-maintenance wildflower meadow.

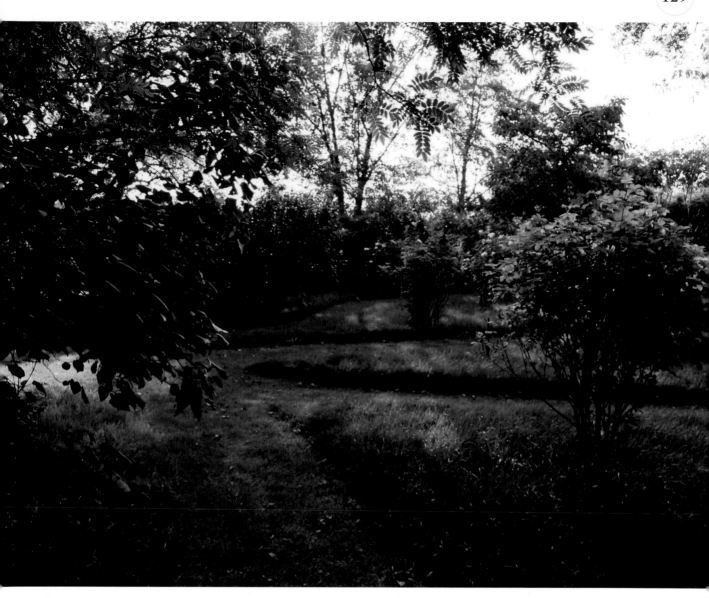

not harm them. Any unwanted thugs can be removed through weeding, or by using chemical weedkiller selectively.

Ecolawns, or 'Mown Green Spaces'

If reducing the hours spent tending the lawn appeals but you still want a short and highly useable grassy area, an ecolawn is a good solution. This is the approach used in HRH The Prince of Wales's garden at Highgrove House, where the term 'mown green spaces'—used in pointed contrast to 'lawns'—is especially apt, as no cultural elements aside from mowing are imposed. In this garden, a cylinder (reel) mower leaves bold stripes in its wake, and cuttings are always removed for composting. The lawn remains green even during very dry periods despite thin, free-draining soil, and this is wholly due to the presence of a tapestry of herbs, many of which have subtle yet attractive flowers.

To achieve a similar effect, you may need to initially carry out the selective weeding regime described in the Wildflower Meadows section. For a good balance of herbs among the grasses you should try to remove the cuttings, although if your soil is poor initially you may get away with using a time-saving mulching mower instead.

Longer grass, mown every three weeks or so during the growing season, looks informal and relaxed but never wild or unkempt.

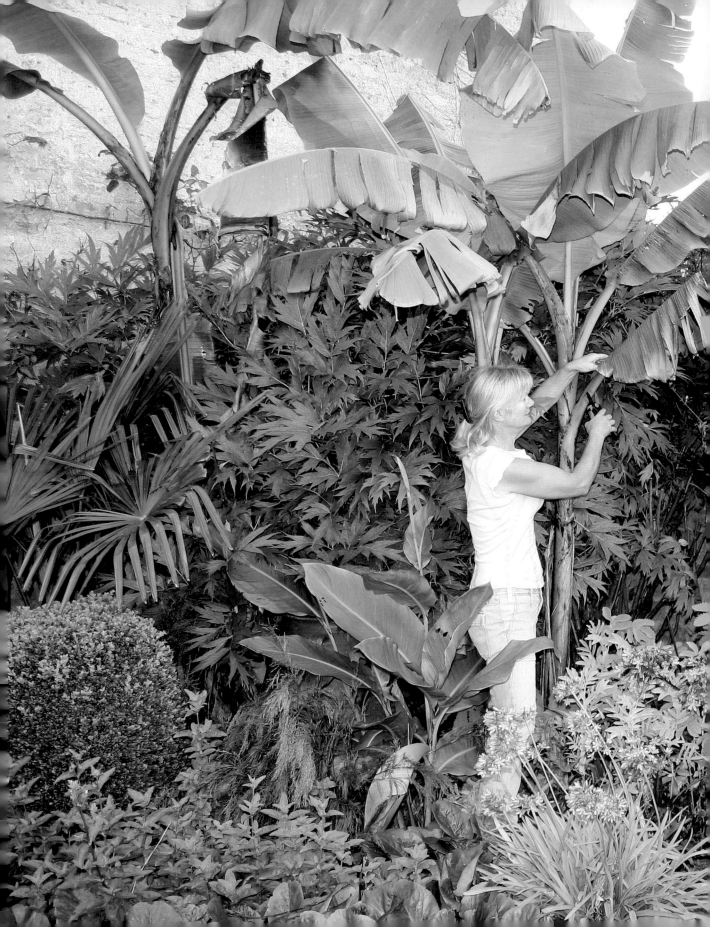

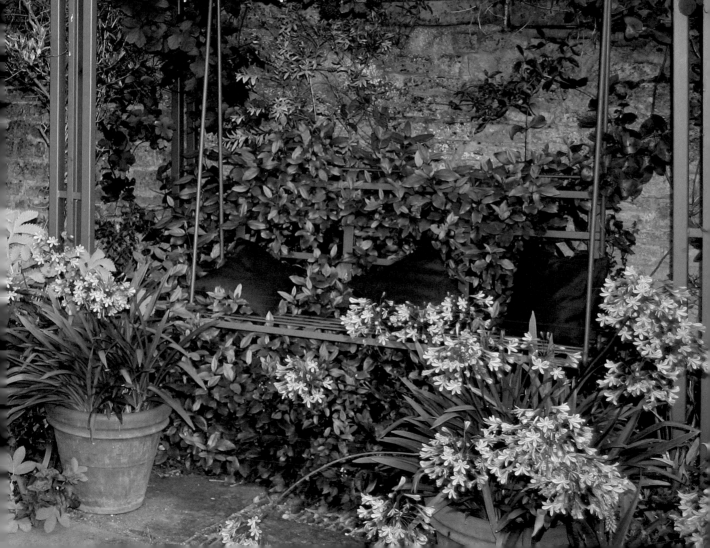

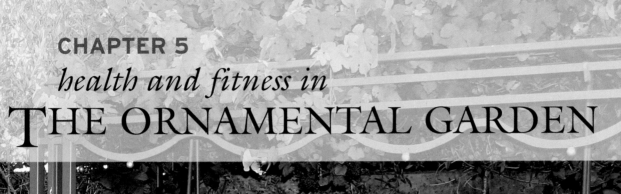

health and fitness in
THE ORNAMENTAL GARDEN

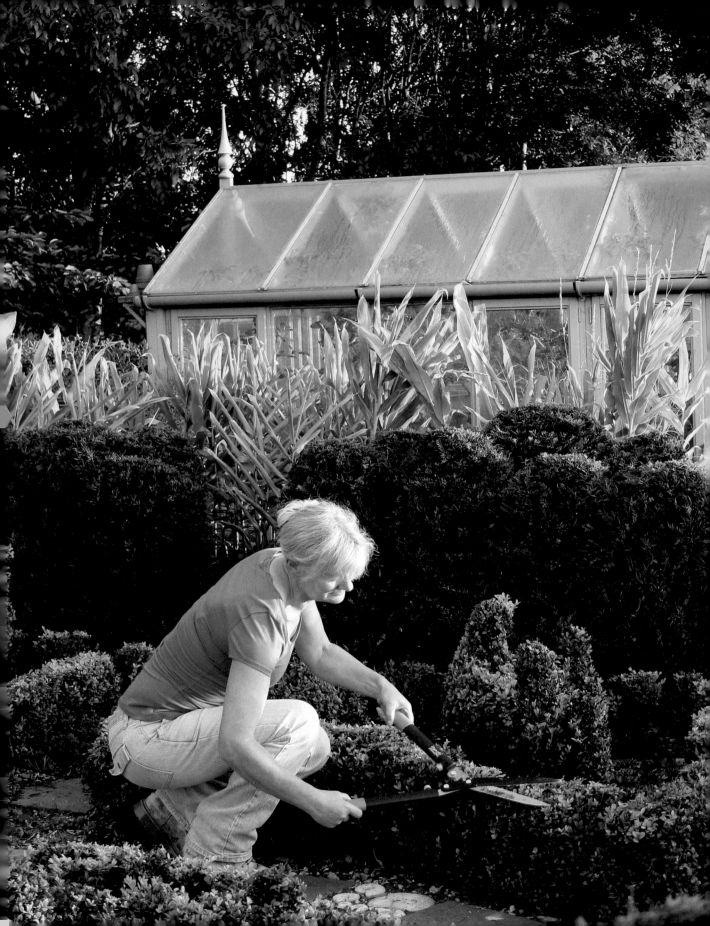

WE ADD PLANTS to our gardens because they enrich the way in which we experience the space. Borders beautify the garden, softening buildings and imbuing the area with fragrance, lushness, texture, and colour. The structural and aesthetic qualities of trees and hedges allow us to personalize our gardens; they serve as focal points, divide a sprawling area into welcoming 'outdoor rooms', and screen gardens to provide privacy and emphasize the most appealing features of the house and the outdoor space. As we select, grow, and nurture plants, they change continuously, keeping us focused and motivated.

To ensure your plantings bring satisfaction and reduce the likelihood of stress and frustration, it is vital to be realistic about the maintenance levels that various planting schemes require, and to create plantings that will thrive with the amount of time and effort you are prepared to devote to them. Some borders, composed of just a few species planted en masse or some ground cover, are so low-maintenance that they virtually care for themselves.

Whether you are aiming for a low-maintenance planting scheme or an intricate flower border, the maintenance demands that the plantings present will inspire you to be active—and as you will be creating something that is aesthetically interesting and/or artistically expressive, you may find that time flies by while you are working in the fresh air. In this chapter, we will explore an array of options for beautifying the garden through various planting schemes and styles, as well as strategies for avoiding frustration and making the garden as successful as possible even when time is limited.

These 'nests' of low box hedging surround a variety of clipped green 'birds'. Ground cover composed of house leeks (*Sempervivum calcareum*) forms the bedding layer. This planting requires cutting twice a year in addition to basic weeding.

Establishing Borders

Although borders are lovely, some gardeners find them daunting as the routine demands of planting, pruning, watering, and feeding can be difficult to get right. Regardless of how well you understand the conditions in your garden, plants can be unpredictable, and finding the right plant for the right place can require considerable effort. Borders give you a valuable chance to be both active and creative in the garden, and all of the thought and planning that they require can really keep you on your toes.

Planning your plantings around the amount of time you want to spend tending to them is key. If your schedule is busy, you can still cultivate a rewarding garden; a low-maintenance planting pattern involving just a handful of high-performance, robust plants may be your best option. Having said that, if you can devote just a few more hours a month to increase the interest levels through more intricate planting schemes, this will add appeal to the garden and provide an incentive for you to stay active. Weeding, which involves a good range of movements (bending, squatting, and kneeling) provides an excuse for regularly stretching your body into rarely used positions—and it eats up calories, too. If you are tentative about being too ambitious with your planting plans, you can always start simply and then diversify as you gain confidence.

MAKING A NEW BORDER FROM LAWN

If you are establishing a new border in the garden, it is important to first take time to lay the groundwork. Although it may be tempting to start planting right away, proper preparation at the outset will save you time and reduce the likelihood of encountering problems at a later stage.

Removing Existing Grass

When removing existing grass to implement a new border, some gardeners are reluctant to resort to chemicals. However, when faced with the challenging task of removing grass, using a translocated herbicide such as glyphosate is an extremely effective and user-friendly way to get the job done. This type of chemical breaks down quickly, does not leach, and is locked up by the soil quite rapidly. By using it in the early stages to get borders up and running and to remove problematic perennial weeds, you can save yourself years of aggravating battle. (If you apply it in colder months when the grass or weeds are not growing rapidly it takes longer—perhaps a few weeks—to work, but it will still be effective.)

An organic alternative would be to cover the area with black polythene until the grass has died right back. Perennial grasses and weeds may yellow off quite quickly, but their roots will still be alive, so it may be necessary to keep the ground covered for several months or even a year. Alternatively, you could lift the turf, but this is hard work and removes the valuable top layer of organic matter and topsoil. It also exposes new weed seeds (in the new top layer of soil) to light—and as soon as this happens, germination may occur. This method may well not remove perennial weeds, either.

To Dig or Not to Dig?

When placing plants in a new flower border where existing grass is present, the first instinct of so many gardeners is to start digging. However, this is not always the best option; at times it can even be counterproductive.

Digging will almost certainly increase the number of perennial weeds in the border. When you dig over soil, you are inadvertently chopping up the roots of perennial weeds, so you may well be propagating and spreading them. What's more, when you dig you risk inadvertently disturbing the myriad of creepy crawlies, beneficial fungi, soil microorganisms, and worms that live beneath the soil's surface. For these reasons, it is not always best to automatically begin digging.

On the other hand, there are times when digging is necessary. For instance, it is essential when you are making a planting hole, breaking up a soil pan, or moving a

Digging can be strenuous work. It is best to keep the digging action close to your body and apply leverage with your foot.

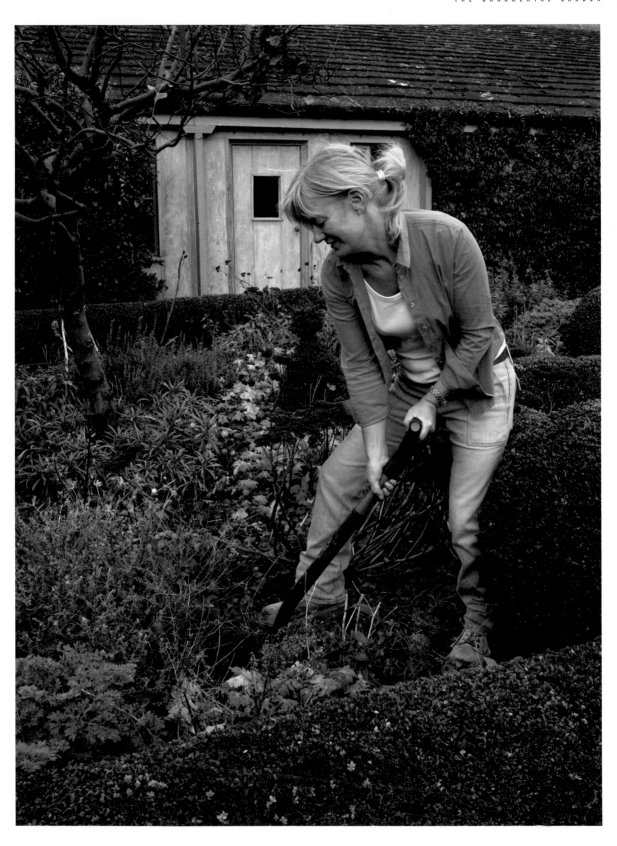

Establishing Borders

mature plant. Most plants do not require a vast pit; the hole for each plant should be just marginally bigger than the plant's root ball, container, or roots, assuming that the soil at the base of it is of decent quality. If you discover a layer of stones or clay, then dig out the most obstructive to ensure that your plant will have drainage and soil at its base. Then, add some compost to the bottom of the hole and around the plant as you place it in the ground.

To increase the fertility and improve the structure of a thin soil, add some good-quality compost to the surface; an abundant supply will increase the worm population tenfold in three years. A healthy worm population can transform soil, aerating it and incorporating humus and organic matter without causing damage.

Digging Safely

Digging the soil is strenuous work. If performed correctly, it works all of your muscle groups; if done incorrectly, though, all the bending and twisting it involves can inflict stress on your lower back and cause injury. To avoid injuring yourself through digging, be sure to warm up beforehand. You should also start slowly, and take regular breaks.

As much as possible, your abdominal muscles should be engaged: picture them staying lifted and strong, absorbing the strenuous impact of the digging action as your back remains upright and supported. Try to practise ambidexterity by alternating sides so that the rotational force on your spine comes from both directions. Along with your abdominal muscles, your quadriceps, hamstrings, and buttocks should be hard at work, while your trunk, shoulders, and arms should take responsibility for shifting the soil. It is best to keep the action close to your body.

The spade you use should be sharp enough to slice the soil and the correct length for your body; the handle should come up to about waist height as this will encourage your back to stay neutral and enable you to apply a greater leverage with your foot when lifting up the soil.

Planting

The next step is to place your plants in the soil. If you opt to propagate these plants yourself (through cuttings, seed, or division) grow them on in hoarding borders until you obtain the quantity and size you require. To make life easier, you can plant through a membrane or use a weed-suppressing mulch; either way, make sure the soil is free of perennial weeds before planting.

Container-grown plants are often on the dry side. Immersing the plant's pot in a bucket of water for a few minutes will moisten the plant far more effectively than just watering the top of the pot. Before you put the plant in the hole, it is often worthwhile to pull off the top ¼ in. (6 mm) of compost on the pot, as this is often full of hairy bittercress seeds. Then, tease out the plant's roots if necessary.

Unless the quality of the soil is poor, it is not necessary to add fertilizer to the planting hole. Instead, it can be added in the form of a mulch or top dressing, where the worms can distribute it into the soil and the rain can wash it down to the roots. Nutrients at the base of the planting hole tend to leach through the soil before the plant has time to tap its roots into it.

A mulch of gravel over the top layer of soil will suppress most annual weeds, although perennial weeds will still need to be removed.

CONSIDER THE WEATHER

As a general rule, it is best to avoid planting on rainy days. Although soil stays much drier under turf than when it is bare of vegetation, it is far better for the soil if you do not work it, dig it, or trample on it unless it is fairly dry. Beautifully structured, brown crumbly soil can quickly become compacted and airless if you garden on it when it is wet.

You will soon notice the difference: in dry periods, the soil will crack into hard blocks, and in wet periods it puddles, does not drain, and become a ghastly surface for growing plants. It really pays off to be patient and wait for a series of fine, non-rainy days before planting. If it is a little damp, it is a good idea to spread out some broad wood planks in the garden on which to work as you carry out your planting.

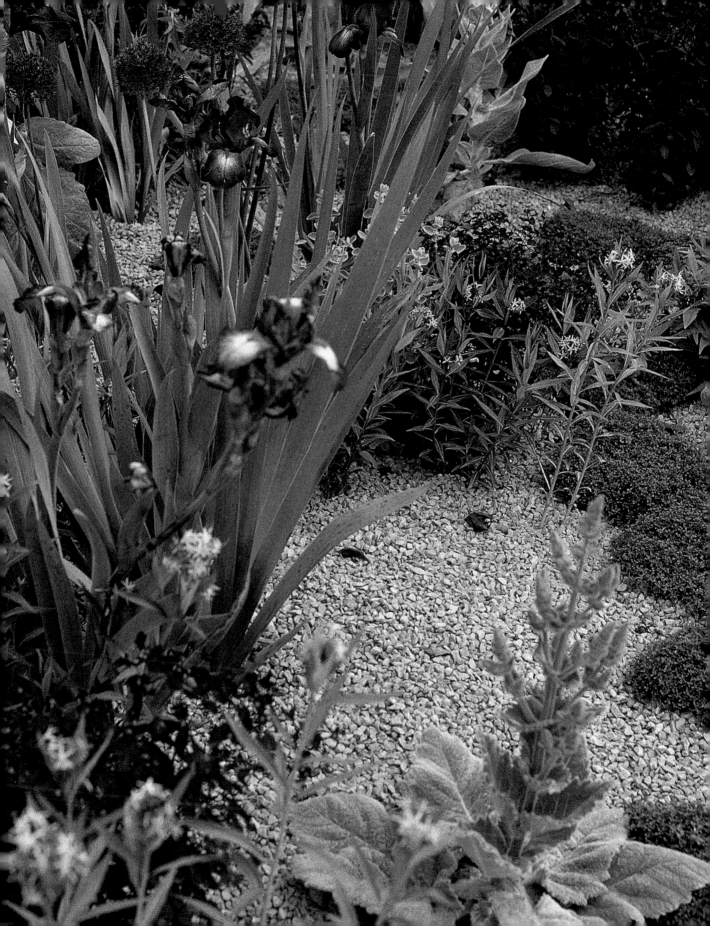

Border Planting Schemes

Depending on the type of planting scheme you choose, maintenance levels can vary tremendously. A simply planted area with drifts of colour may well be able to thrive with a single maintenance visit each month (or, in some cases, each year), while a diverse, elaborate border requires seemingly constant attention. As a general rule, the more species of plants you decide to include, the more difficult the maintenance will be.

LOW-MAINTENANCE BORDERS
When it comes to low-maintenance borders, gardeners have a range of options. The simplest borders require far less maintenance than a mown lawn does, and when carefully planned they can be highly attractive.

Massed Blocks
The simplest kind of border involves using just one, or very few, types of plants in a massed block. To keep maintenance demands as low as possible, it is essential to remove all the perennial weeds and the majority of the annual weed seed burden first, and then plant densely. You may want to use mulch (or a fabric membrane plus mulch) at the time of planting.

Ground Cover
Ground cover can be supremely low-maintenance, especially if only a few different species of plant are used. For instance if you plant a sheet of creeping comfrey (*Symphytum* 'Hidcote Blue') under a block of trees it dispenses with the need to mow between the trees, and once established, this ground cover would probably take less than one day per year to maintain. Ivy (species of *Hedera*), vigorous ferns, and periwinkle (species of *Vinca*) are also good options as they yield satisfying results with minimal maintenance. These plants usually spread through root suckers, or stolons; once the individual plants meet up, the need to weed becomes minimal. Simply carry out a quick check once every month during the growing season to see if any weeds have emerged.

MOWING MARGINS

In any flower border, one of the most difficult parts to look after is the junction between grass and planting. If you design long, thin, rectangular borders set among grass, it will significantly increase your labour input. A mowing margin will counteract this, stopping the grass from colonizing the flower beds and adding structure.

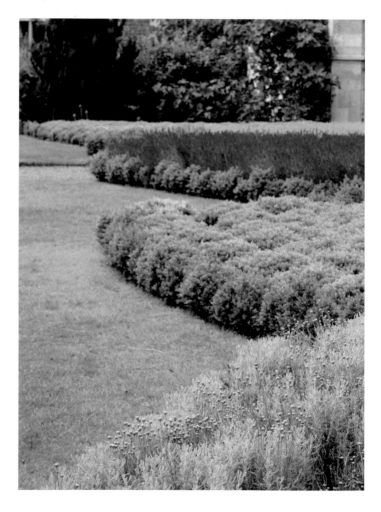

Large blocks of certain plants look fabulous en masse. Lavender looks particularly attractive when planted in this way, and the compact hebe gives good winter structure.

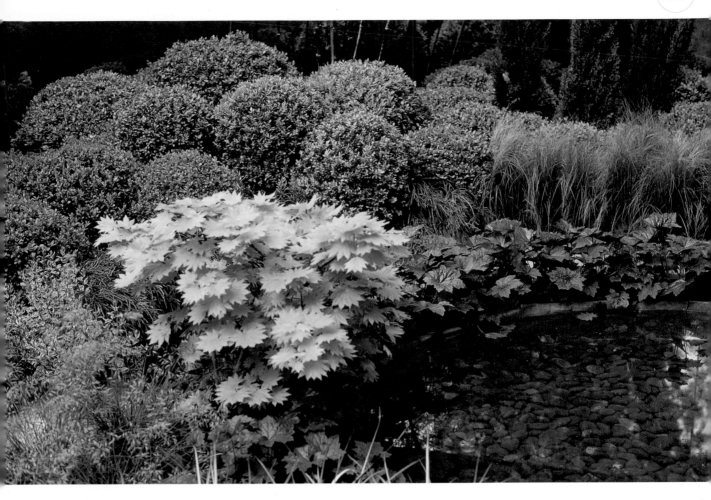

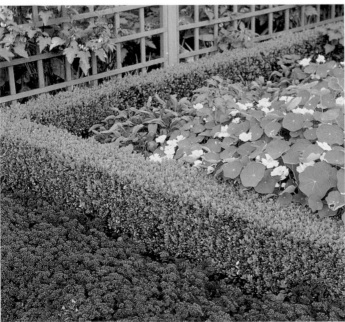

LEFT: You can afford to be bold with colour on hard surfaces when it is broken up by planting rather than in big solid blocks. Here a painted trellis, an edging of box, and the use of evergreen plants within the planting keep this mainly green-and-purple-themed border looking colourful all year round. The trellis is painted to highlight the colour theme.

ABOVE: Even in the winter, this planting provides visual impact. The cluster of differently sized box balls and the heuchera make strong year-round statements.

Border Planting Schemes

When some woody ground cover plants grow old they become less leafy, upping the likelihood of weeds invading the patch. The low-growing cotoneasters in particular tend to thin out and grow bald as they age. It is easy to regenerate most over-mature ground cover plants, however: simply cut them back to 2- to 4-in. (5- to 10-cm) stumps, and then give them a feed and a mulch.

Fabric Membrane Planting

Using fabric membranes with ground cover plants or shrubs can result in an extremely low-maintenance border, as the fabric membranes suppress weeds. (On commercial planting schemes that thrive on one maintenance visit a year, it is normal to use vigorous, tough plants that cover ground quickly through a fabric, and then to hide the fabric with a thick layer of coarse grade mulch.)

Choose the smaller, easier shrubs such as potentilla or euonymus, or taller shrubs such as large shrub roses, cotoneasters, or *Viburnum tinus*. Place four plants per square yard (or square metre) with clumps, drifts or blocks of the same species planted together so that one species is less likely to out-compete another. Herbaceous plants that increase by spreading sideways do not work well in this situation, and keen gardeners would find it frustrating not to be able to easily dig and add plants as they wanted. However, in certain situations membrane planting is invaluable.

Massed Blocks with Filling

Another easy but satisfying option is to choose a long-flowering plant and surround it with plants that offer year-round interest. For instance, massed *Erigeron karvinskianus*, edged by low box hedging

BELOW: **Strong structural beds lined with box and filled with one type of plant simplify maintenance demands.**

BELOW RIGHT: **Two simple, identically planted beds both feature a small ornamental tree with a box plinth, a sheet of *Stachys byzantina*, and an outer informal hedge of *Teucrium ×lucidrys*.**

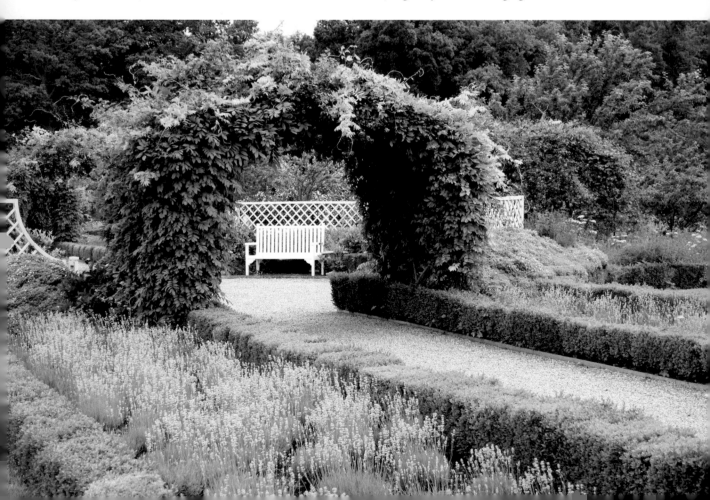

and studded with a few simple bits of topiary, is a sound option. The 'daisies' flower for a good ten months each year, and the hedging, topiary, and foliage remain attractive when the flowering season has passed.

Erigeron karvinskianus is probably one of the most long-performing options for the 'filling'. Simple alternatives include herbaceous geraniums especially *Geranium* 'Jolly Bee' and 'Rozanne', which are both excellent blues that flower from June to November. *Teucrium ×lucidrys* is a neat evergreen with mauve flowers that last for a long time.

Stachys byzantina 'Big Ears' forms dense sheets of silver, grey-felted foliage. It is a useful, permanently attractive low-level plant that is ideal for planting around the base of topiary.

If you covet more colour but still want to keep maintenance levels low, certain low roses such as *Rosa* 'Marie Pavic', *Rosa* 'Flower Carpet', and *Rosa* 'The Fairy' are easy, long-flowering, and tough.

EASY SELF-SEEDERS

The following are all easy-to-grow self-seeding annuals, self-seeding biennials, or short-lived perennials:

Digitalis purpurea (common foxglove): white, crimson, pale yellow, or mauve

Verbascum bombyciferum 'Polarsommer' (mullein): pale yellow

Hesperis matronalis (sweet rocket): white or pale pink

Lunaria annua and *L. rediviva*: white and purple

Matthiola incana (stock): pink, white, or purple, with evergreen foliage

Lychnis coronaria (Dusty Miller): strong magenta-pink

Lychnis coronaria 'Alba': white

Verbena bonariensis: purple

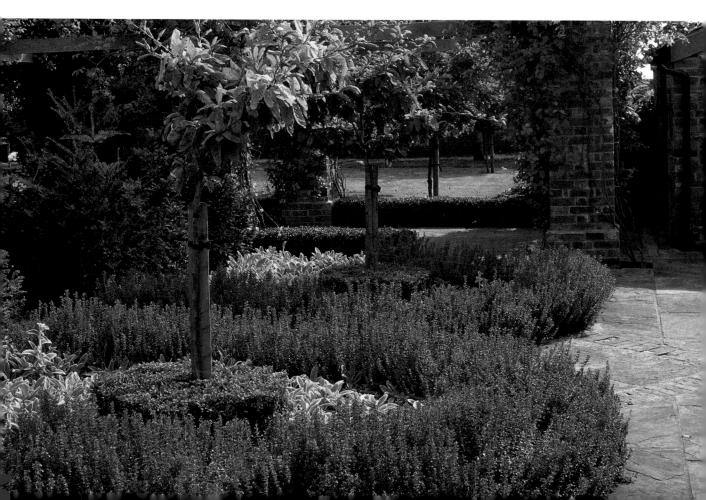

Border Planting Schemes

WATERING WISELY

Keep in mind that new plants will require water for at least the first few months after planting, during their first growing season. (Roses are a special case, as they benefit from extra water throughout their first two years after planting.) Watering should ideally be carried out in the evening rather than in the morning, as this allows the water to be soaked up overnight before the sun comes out.

As a general rule, you should add larger volumes of water once in a while rather than smaller volumes frequently; this way, you encourage the plants' roots to delve down into the earth, encouraging them to stand on their own roots sooner.

Lack of water, or too much water, are the commonest reasons why new plants fail. When you buy in plants from a nursery, keep in mind that they will have been spoon-fed, and that garden conditions tend to be more hostile than those of the nursery, particularly when it comes to exposure. Keep a regular eye on your new plants; as they say in China, the best manure is the shadow of the gardener. If you are using a mulch (with or without a fabric membrane), the plant must be well watered before the mulch is applied.

If your plants begin to wilt, they may be suffering from drought or overwatering, gently push your fingers down into the soil to see if it feels too wet or too dry.

Carrying Water Cans

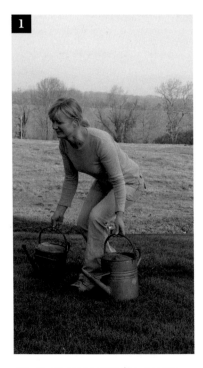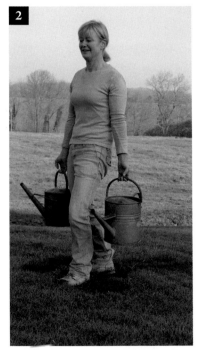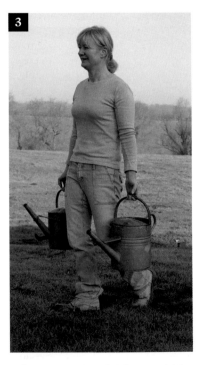

1 If you need to pick the watering cans up from the ground, bend your knees and keep your back straight. Try to distribute the weight evenly between your two hands.

2 Next, stand up straight and pull your lower stomach upwards and inwards. Your spine should be in its neutral position. Relax your shoulders, keeping your shoulder blades pressed down into your back to minimize strain on your shoulders and neck.

3 As you walk, maintain an upright posture and keep your stomach drawn up and in. The weight of the watering cans should be taken on by your abdominal muscles and shoulder blades.

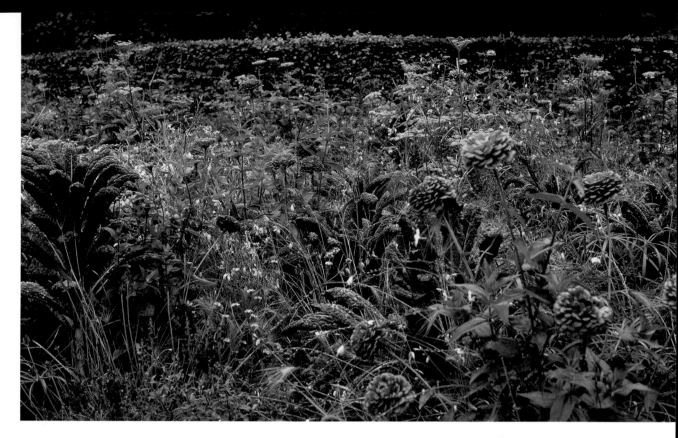

MODERATE-MAINTENANCE BORDERS

If you have slightly more time to devote to garden maintenance, you can create a more elaborate border using a handful of different high-performance plants.

Prairie-style Planting

One option is to use large drifts of perennials in a prairie-style planting. If you have reasonably fertile soil and several square yards (or metres) of space to fill, you can select large, robust perennials that favour your soil conditions, and cultivate generous swathes of these freestyle plantings. Golden rod (*Solidago* species), Joe-Pye weed (*Eupatorium fistulosum*) and coneflowers (*Rudbeckia* species) are popular. To keep maintenance down, make sure the initial soil is clean, and ensure that any cultivars and hybrids are as close to the wild species as possible, as these plants are often more vigorous, and therefore require less cosseting than garden cultivars do. Plant them at close centres—try eight per square yard (or metre)—to ensure that virtually all bare earth is covered as soon as possible. Consider adding ornamental grasses, too.

Large drifts of perennials start to come into their own in midsummer. In late summer they really come to life, and their seedheads will often hold interest until mid or late winter. From the end of winter until late spring, after you have chopped it all down to ground level and before the plants spring back into growth, these areas can look bleak; in places such as England where the climate is gentle, these large expanses of perennials (plus a few grasses) need to be carefully sited, as they can look rather forlorn during these transitional months. On the other hand, in areas with harsher climates, such as northern Japan and parts of North America, this is of no consequence as the area will often be covered by a blanket of snow. The new growth tends to be put on very quickly when spring arrives, making the desolate stage very short-lived.

Patterns Using Distinct Blocks

Designing a scheme with distinct blocks of plants laid out in simple patterns will make interest levels leap up several notches. In the sketches on the next page, four planting schemes are illustrated. In order to keep the blocks distinct, you need to choose a plant's neighbours carefully. Remember that it is often the interface between the different types of plants that causes the required maintenance levels to increase.

Here ephemeral plants including black kale (*Cavolo nero*) and pink dahlias, are mixed up together. This type of planting scheme looks sensational during summertime, but in winter and spring the interest is low.

Border Planting Schemes

Massed Planting Schemes: Four Plans

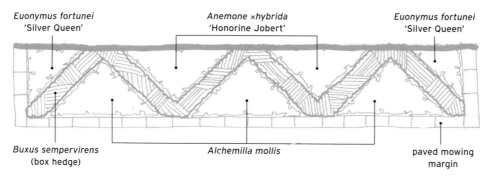

Euonymus fortunei 'Silver Queen'

Anemone ×hybrida 'Honorine Jobert'

Euonymus fortunei 'Silver Queen'

Buxus sempervirens (box hedge)

Alchemilla mollis

paved mowing margin

Here the low box hedge does all the separating for you. The hedging can be designed in many different shapes and patterns such as scallops, blocks or diamonds. You can use paving slabs instead, if you do not want to clip the hedge every year.

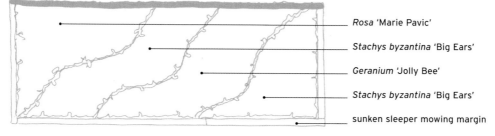

Rosa 'Marie Pavic'

Stachys byzantina 'Big Ears'

Geranium 'Jolly Bee'

Stachys byzantina 'Big Ears'

sunken sleeper mowing margin

In this instance Stachys byzantina 'Big Ears' may start to grow under the low rose, but because their respective canopy heights are at different levels it is not a problem.

bottomless pots planted with topiary

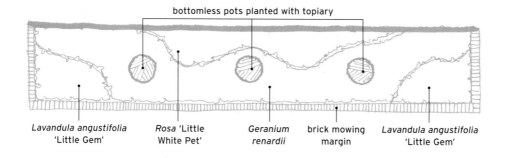

Lavandula angustifolia 'Little Gem'

Rosa 'Little White Pet'

Geranium renardii

brick mowing margin

Lavandula angustifolia 'Little Gem'

This lavender will need cutting back hard after flowering, at least just before late summer, so it can regrow into neat hummocks of foliage to look presentable through the winter. Three bottomless planted pots punctuate the bed.

small specimen tree, e.g. quince (Cydonia oblonga)

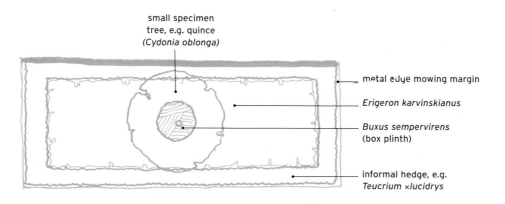

metal edge mowing margin

Erigeron karvinskianus

Buxus sempervirens (box plinth)

informal hedge, e.g. Teucrium ×lucidrys

Placed centrally, this small open-canopied specimen tree adds wonderful three-dimensional appeal. The base of the trunk is surrounded by a low plinth of box, and a mattress of Erigeron karvinskianus, which flowers almost continuously and really lights up the ground.

Planting Density

All of the plants mentioned in the examples on the left are excellent workhorses under most normal soil conditions. However, as often is the case, the grey-leaved plants such as lavender and *Stachys* species should be avoided if your soil is at all heavy or waterlogged. Most of these plants, excluding the roses and hedging, could be planted at a density of eight per square yard (or square metre). Positioned in this way, they would cover the ground quickly, leaving little room for weeds to creep in.

The eventual spread of these plants will be quite extensive—indeed far more than you are allowing with these densities—but to ensure you achieve a stable colony of plants, you should plant at a higher density than you actually need. The small roses could be placed at four or five plants per square yard (or square metre).

Increasing Colour Levels

Using repeated groups of bulbs and self-seeding annuals, biennials, and short-lived perennials can bump up colour levels in your planting scheme without massively increasing the workload. After a few years these plants can become too invasive, but they are fairly easy to thin out through weeding. Placing a few pockets of annuals into the mix makes for more predictable planting schemes but, of course, requires a bit more work; a few clumps of tobacco plants, cosmos, tall white cleomes, or any other favourites will imbue your border with an extra three-month-long colour boost.

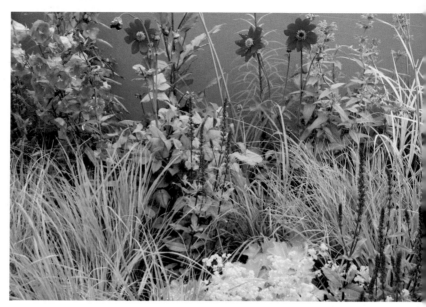

BELOW: Dahlias, salvias, penstemons, and campanulas give summer colour.

BOTTOM: Alliums, chives, and purple castor oil plants add temporary colour boosts.

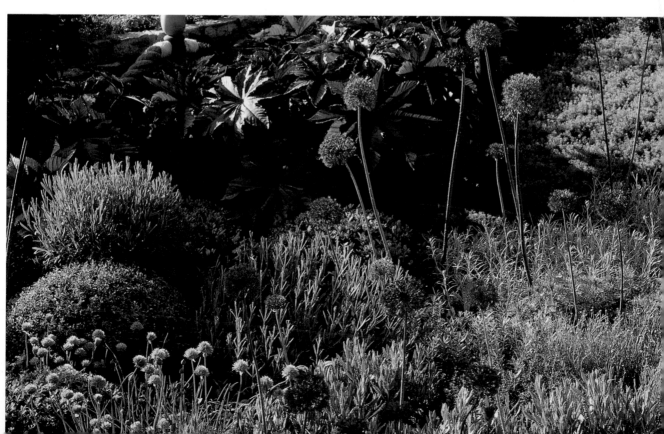

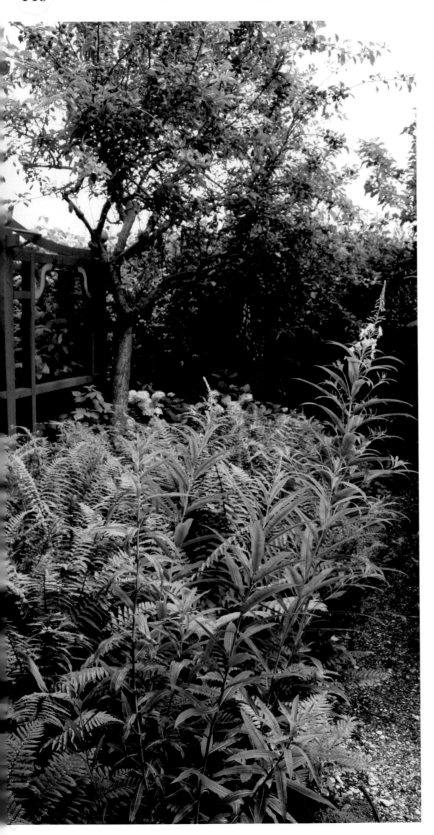

Mixing Permanent and Temporary Plants

Many gardeners enjoy planting with a diverse array of types of plants that have different flowering periods. This keeps the garden looking continuously dynamic, interesting, and alive as it evolves throughout the changing seasons. A wide variety of plants makes for a richer variety of scents, blooms, and foliage.

Caring for a variety of different plants as they jostle side by side in intricate planting schemes requires significant time and attention; for instance, a robust geranium will continuously try to encroach on a more recently planted, less vigorous phlox if this border is not carefully managed. Borders are never static from year to year; rather, the balance is dynamic and what is harmonious one year may well result in a riot the next.

The labour required is not necessarily onerous, but you do need to watch over your plantings and carry out short, regular (often weekly) bursts of activity during the growing season. This may involve deadheading to encourage more flowering, planting in and removing seasonal colour, adding bulbs, and cutting back or clipping vigorous plants. If you spend this extra time you should see real rewards in that your border and the extra regular attention required will keep you active and engaged.

If you need to leave this type of planting to its own devices over several weeks, it should not cause any real problems; when you do return to your maintenance routine, the titivating will take slightly longer. However, recall that is generally unwise to leave weeks between gardening sessions and then jump back into the activities vigorously. If you tackle a range of gardening tasks after a break, be sure to do so gently and warm up beforehand.

This bed was free of weeds prior to planting and then was thickly planted with blocks of various ferns. A few clumps of the white willow herb (*Chamerion angustifolium* 'Album') contrast with the fresh green ferns.

Mixed Planting Schemes: Two Plans

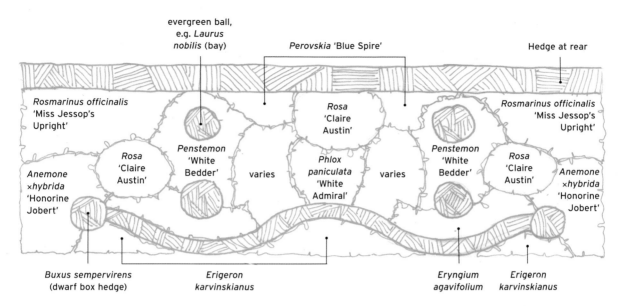

evergreen ball,
e.g. *Laurus
nobilis* (bay)

Perovskia 'Blue Spire'

Hedge at rear

Rosmarinus officinalis
'Miss Jessop's
Upright'

Rosa
'Claire
Austin'

Rosmarinus officinalis
'Miss Jessop's
Upright'

Rosa
'Claire
Austin'

Penstemon
'White
Bedder'

varies

*Phlox
paniculata*
'White
Admiral'

varies

Penstemon
'White
Bedder'

Rosa
'Claire
Austin'

*Anemone
×hybrida*
'Honorine
Jobert'

*Anemone
×hybrida*
'Honorine
Jobert'

Buxus sempervirens
(dwarf box hedge)

*Erigeron
karvinskianus*

*Eryngium
agavifolium*

*Erigeron
karvinskianus*

In the border above, the section that "varies",
flanking the central *Phlox paniculata* 'White
Admiral', could be composed of white wallflowers
(from the genus *Erysimum*) and tulips, then
replaced with a tender perennial like *Salvia indica*
'Indigo Spires', for the summer and autumn.

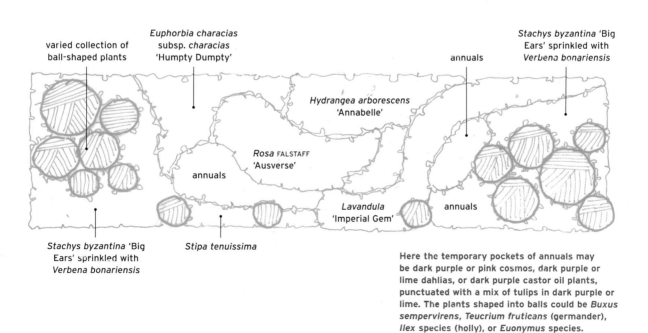

varied collection of
ball-shaped plants

Euphorbia characias
subsp. *characias*
'Humpty Dumpty'

annuals

Stachys byzantina 'Big
Ears' sprinkled with
Verbena bonariensis

Hydrangea arborescens
'Annabelle'

Rosa FALSTAFF
'Ausverse'

annuals

Lavandula
'Imperial Gem'

annuals

Stachys byzantina 'Big
Ears' sprinkled with
Verbena bonariensis

Stipa tenuissima

Here the temporary pockets of annuals may
be dark purple or pink cosmos, dark purple or
lime dahlias, or dark purple castor oil plants,
punctuated with a mix of tulips in dark purple or
lime. The plants shaped into balls could be *Buxus
sempervirens*, *Teucrium fruticans* (germander),
Ilex species (holly), or *Euonymus* species.

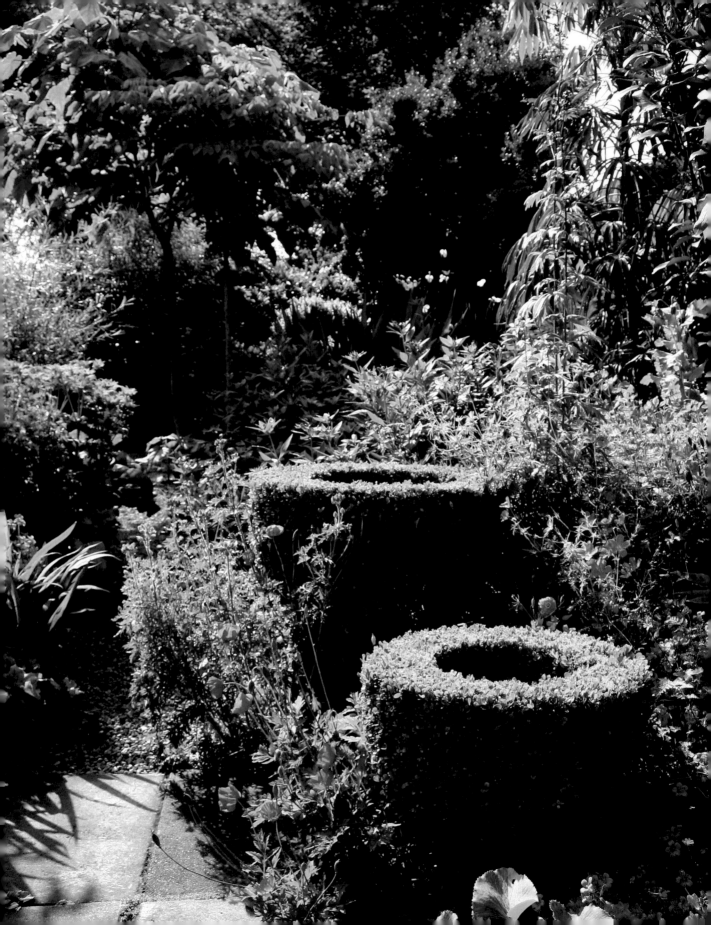

In both of these schemes a basic strong nucleus of evergreens, shrubs, roses, and perennials has been 'zapped up' by injecting temporary colour of tender perennials, dahlias, bulbs, or annuals. A major perk of this mixed planting approach is that although the basic planting is fairly constant and stable, the annuals that you add to the mix can change. One year you may want to plant bold groups of the pungent pink *Dahlia* 'Fascination'; then, the next year you can add a tropical bent with clumps of orange cannas, and the following year airy groups of the tall, tender *Salvia* 'Indigo Spires' might steal the show.

Avoid the pitfall of using many different kinds of plants simply for the sake of doing so; even on the most intricate extensive borders, a limited palette of different plants used in bold repeated clumps will hold interest, especially if you increase the colour levels with removable 'add-ins'.

Keep in mind that borders tend to be viewed from certain vantage points. If a long, rectangular border is mostly seen from the narrow end, you can get away with a few gaps and errors in the middle zones, whereas the ends will need special attention to ensure they look as attractive as possible. When you fill in the gaps during the dormant season, you often forget that many gaps have been filled with copious foliage during past summers. Keeping photographic records will help you to stay on track.

LEFT: In Helen Dillon's Dublin garden, the soft forms of the annuals and perennials contrast with the box 'pots'. These intriguing shapes were converted from box balls.

CHOOSING HIGH-PERFORMANCE STRUCTURAL PLANTS

Structural plants form the backbone of the border; at least 30% of your border could be comprised of them. In a group of borders surrounding one space, or perhaps in a large border, you may decide to use five different plants or clumps of structural plants repeatedly. (To lower the maintenance burden, increase the evergreen/grey structural plant component of your garden's planting scheme to around 50%).

The vast majority of these plants will require annual clipping or pruning in order to stay in shape. I suggest doing this in early autumn, when tasks in the garden are generally less hectic. If you want to reduce the time spent clipping and trimming, choose the slower-growing plants; often they take a few years to form large, shapely specimens. If you start off with small plants, you can fill in the areas around them with cheap, disposable, easily propagated plants such as *Alchemilla mollis*, *Vinca* species or herbaceous geraniums in the interim.

Certain structural plants are consistently good performers under a wide range of garden conditions. For instance, *Buxus sempervirens* is useful as hedging and topiary, and lends itself well to being cloud-pruned. The fast-growing *Teucrium fruticans* (germander) looks fabulous when kept lightly shaped, and *Hebe rakaiensis*, coloured bright green, is easily propagated and fast growing. *Euonymus fortunei* 'Silver Queen' is easy to clip into balls or mounds, and can grow in dry or shady situations.

Brachyglottis (formerly *Senecio*) Dunedin Group 'Sunshine' is fast growing and tolerant of many conditions. Some choose to remove the yellow flowers and shape the shrub up annually, but consider using *Brachyglottis monroi* over *Brachyglottis greyii*, as it is more compact and its unusual flowers are less conspicuous.

Lavandula angustifolia 'Imperial Gem' is one of the best lavenders, as it is long-flowering and produces good winter foliage. It requires a well-drained soil and must be cut back by the beginning of late summer so new growth forms for winter appeal. *Osmanthus delavayi* has white flowers and adds great sense of structure to a space. Other sound choices are *Pittosporum tobira* (which can be tender) and *Pittosporum tenuifolium* 'Abbotsbury Gold'. If you have the patience, you can form great shapes with *Ilex aquifolium* (holly) and *Laurus nobilis* (bay).

When establishing a box hedge, bare root plants are less expensive than container-grown plants to buy and will often grow on quicker and better. They are easy to root from cuttings that can be rooted in seed trays in early autumn. It is possible to cram in a good seventy-five cuttings per tray. Ideally, they should be stored in a greenhouse, cold frame, or sheltered place outside, and by late in the following spring you should find that many are beginning to root well.

Border Planting Schemes

HIGH-MAINTENANCE BORDERS

Many famous borders in well-known gardens are an eclectic mix of bulbs, perennials, annuals, shrubs, roses, tender perennials, and even more. Often there are literally hundreds of different species used, and in the most celebrated and eye-catching of borders the roster of plants tends to vary continuously.

If you are a plantaholic and love playing around with your plants by staking, deadheading, clipping, and moving them, following this style will be immensely rewarding. To avoid disappointment, it is important to make sure you have significant time to devote to the planting schemes.

You can manipulate the flowering time and height of many perennials by cutting them back before they flower. This will delay their flowering time and usually results in more plantiful yet slightly smaller flowers.

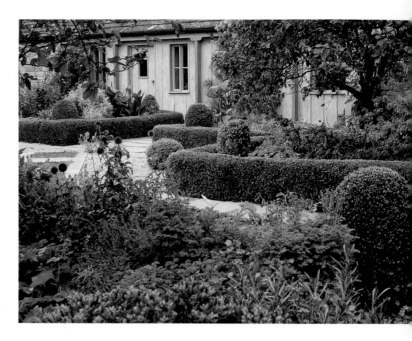

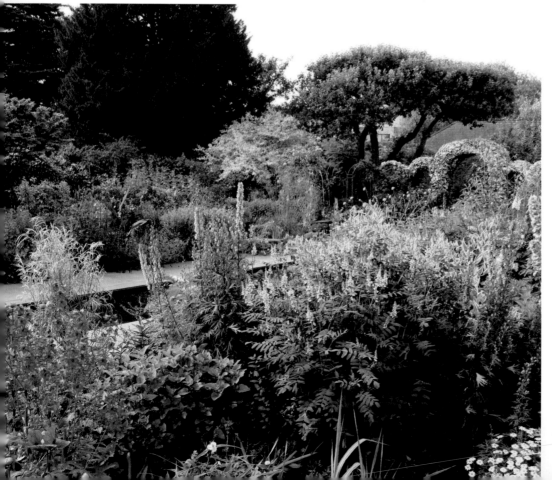

ABOVE: In the borders around my courtyard, an abundance of shaped evergreen plants coupled with the structural form of the quince trees gives permanent structure. Large blocks of easy, long-flowering perennials and shrub roses provide very long-lasting colour and small pockets of annuals, bulbs, and tender perennials add a bit of higher-maintenance drama.

LEFT: These fabulous borders are in Helen Dillon's garden in Dublin. They contain a mix of many different plants and are pepped up with different bulbs, annuals, and tender perennials through the year. In addition, they are regularly deadheaded, cut back, and generally nurtured to keep them looking fantastic through the changing seasons.

Weed Control

Keeping weeds at bay is essential to the success of any planting scheme. Although hand weeding may seem laborious, it does give you an excuse to spend time enjoying your plants at extremely close quarters. It is also an excellent way to exercise (provided you do it the right way), and once you start weeding, the time tends to fly by and you may not even realize that you are engaging in quite strenuous, physical exercise in the rejuvenating fresh air.

It is crucial to stay on top of the weed situation rather than letting it get out of hand, as this can be a source of stress; it can be frustrating to tackle sprawling areas full of vigorous weeds that are spitting out their seeds the moment you disturb them. To keep weeds under control, it helps to know your weeds' habits, which can vary widely.

For best results, be sure to clean new borders of all perennial weeds before you plant. If you can get into a routine of regularly inspecting all areas of the garden—perhaps incorporating this into a simple fitness routine as you jog through your garden's pathways each morning—then you will notice new pockets of weeds in their infancy so that you can deal with them before they set seed and spread their wares.

Some plants are so invasive that they will happily colonize vast tracts of space, leaving little room for more reticent types. Many of these most raucous plants are imports which have no predators to control them. Japanese knotweed (*Fallopia japonica*), for example, is tolerated in its native Japan (some people even eat its young shoots). Yet since this plant was introduced into British gardens, it has been overly invasive, spreading rapidly from garden to garden and even pushing up through concrete roads. British gardeners find it difficult to control even with glyphosate. Conversely, in Japan, the English dandelion (*Taraxacum officinale*) is prone to taking over gardens, and is very difficult to control.

Certain weeds, such as groundsel (*Senecio vulgaris*) stagger their germination period so seedlings come up virtually in any month. Try to pull them out before they flower, as the plants can flower and set seed in just five weeks—and if you hoe it off in flower it often carries on and sets seed even when the parent plant looks fairly desiccated. A single plant will produce over a thousand seeds!

Other weeds have explosive seedpods that can fire seeds up to 3 ft. (90 cm)—often just at the moment you reach out to grab them from under your favourite plant. One example is the annual hairy bittercress (*Cardamine hirsute*), the seeds of which are often found in the compost on top of the containers you buy at garden centres. It is worth removing the very surface compost and burying it in the base of the planting hole so that any weed seeds present do not receive enough light to germinate. In seed form, this explosive weed is virtually invisible, while the young plants appear small and harmless and the leaves are tasty in salads. However, be warned: it is highly tenacious, and if you turn your back on it when it looks innocuous you will regret it only a few weeks later.

The saying 'one year's seeding is seven years' weeding' is an understatement in many cases. The annual sow thistle (*Sonchus* species) can produce up to twenty-five thousand seeds in its short life, and the seeds of an opium poppy can last for a century or so. Be careful not to toss weed seeds onto compost heaps as this will encourage their proliferation—instead, put them in a bucket of water so that they rot. They can then be placed onto the compost heap.

SUPPLEMENTARY WEED CONTROL FOR CHALLENGING AREAS

In very challenging areas, you often need to adopt more aggressive strategies against weeds. With existing beds that are very weedy, adding a thick layer of mulch helps enormously with annual weeds. Perennial weeds, however, are especially difficult to eradicate effectively and when they are intertwined with plants it becomes virtually impossible. Because they spread underground, you invariably chop up the

Weed Control

HAND WEEDING

Although it has a reputation of being laborious, hand weeding gives you the opportunity to move your body through a wide range of great exercise positions. Hand weeding in gravel (shown below) is even more satisfying than most weeding because the weeds usually pull out very easily, provided the area has not been left bone dry for weeks.

Weeding is one maintenance action that should be carried out as regularly as possible. If you leave it for too long, it becomes a real chore because there is so much to do. Use the need to weed as an excuse for spending ten minutes in the sunshine.

To avoid strain to your joints and muscles, take a break from hand weeding every fifteen minutes to stroll around the garden, or practice squats or spine curls. It is important that you avoid staying in one position for too long; if your back or knee joints start to feel uncomfortable, get out of the position you are in and move around or do some stretching. If you suffer from knee problems or have a joint replacement, it will not be possible to manoeuvre your body into these positions for weeding. You might try using padded kneelers.

Weeding while kneeling can place undue stress on your hands and wrists so try and keep them as straight as possible. On the other hand, this is a lovely position for your back, as it is relatively easy for your spine to stay in neutral, avoiding strain.

POSITION ONE: **Squatting**

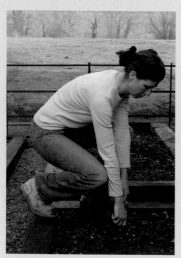

Begin by positioning yourself as close to the weeds as possible, bending your knees and keeping your back in its neutral position. Avoid neck strain by keeping your shoulder blades down and in (picture them pointing towards the centre of your back). Use your shoulder blade muscles to weed. As you shift your weight onto your toes, keep your back in a neutral position, working from your shoulder blades all the while.

POSITION TWO: **Bending**

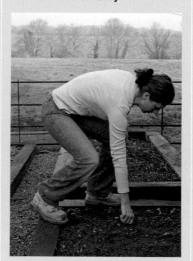

You can also weed while bending over. Your knees should be bent and your back in neutral. Try to crouch by moving your hips, rather than your back. Remember to engage your lower abdominal muscles throughout.

POSITION THREE: **Kneeling**

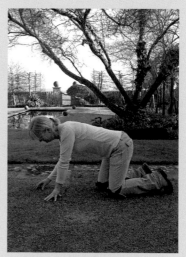

A further option is to weed by kneeling on your hands and knees. It is important to have something to kneel on, whether this is a pad or kneelers built into your trousers. Try to keep your back in its neutral position. As in the squatting position, your shoulder blades should be held down and in towards the middle of your back. Your elbows should be softly bent.

underground roots or rhizomes when you attempt to dig them out, which propagates them even more.

Most dedicated organic gardeners would agree that manual removal manages the situation as opposed to removing the culprits entirely. It is equally difficult to manually remove weeds from large stretches of gravel that are in close proximity to areas that generate masses of weed seeds.

If you are faced with these challenging areas, chemical weed control may be the most efficient option. You may wish to mix and match chemical and hand weeding, by hand weeding where you can and then carrying out a spot treatment of large areas using a knapsack sprayer.

For gravelly areas, gardeners who are wary of using harsh chemicals should consider using glyphosate, a translocated herbicide that kills perennial and annual weeds. Although it would require you to apply more treatments per year than a residual chemical would, a non-residual herbicide like glyphosate may be more environmentally friendly, as smaller amounts of less persistent chemicals are being sprayed. Moreover, if you were using a residual chemical, you would broadcast it over an entire area; by using a non-residual herbicide such as glyphosate you have more control over which plants you eradicate so that you can decide which self-seeders, if any, you want to retain.

Another effective way to control weeds in gravel is by continual trampling of any areas where you want to discourage weeds. If you slightly alter the route you normally take around the garden, this can have a significant effect on weed populations. Also, if you can find time to rake your gravel regularly, this movement helps to control weeds. (It is also good routine exercise, and keeps the gravel looking fresh.)

If you have large gravelly areas and want to be totally organic, however, a flame gun is an extremely popular and effective approach. The heat it emits will kill some of the weed seeds on the surface of the gravel as well as existing weeds, reducing the amount of treatments needed to around four or five each year.

If you are not averse to using a herbicide in your toolbox, dichlobenil (often marketed as Caseron G4 Weed Barrier) is highly effective when applied to borders as a granule during the winter. It will suppress weeds for most of the growing season and works well in areas with established shrubs, trees, and roses.

Many owners of larger gardens depend on using it for extensive shrubberies, under hedgerows, and around trees. It will suppress and kill most annual and perennial weed growth (including Japanese knotweed and field horsetail but excluding bramble) for a good six months. It is most effective when applied to a clean soil, as opposed to one with overwintering weeds, although it will still work to a fair degree if this is not feasible. If you are growing perennials in your borders, or have just planted your shrubs, it will affect them adversely; dichlobenil should only be used for plants that are established and shrubby in nature.

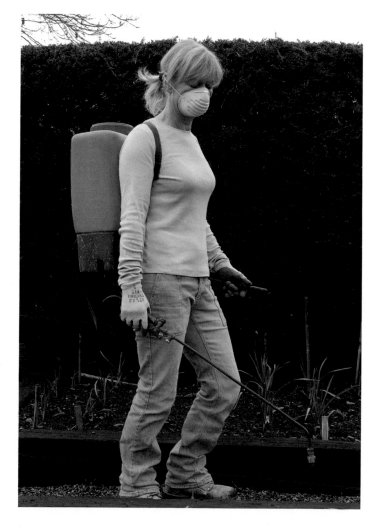

Spraying requires that you wear various safety accessories, depending on which chemicals you are using. Here, a face mask and gloves are worn. The short, taut straps of the knapsack allow you to stand upright, with your back in neutral, drawing your lower abdominals up and in. Your shoulder blades should be set down towards the middle of your back so that you avoid straining your neck.

Designing with Trees and Hedges

Despite being less obviously decorative than their flowery counterparts, trees and hedges are the unsung heroes of the ornamental garden. Wildly diverse and highly malleable, they are the tools that let you structure your space in a way that works for you. Through clever use of trees and hedging, you can frame a beautiful view, create interesting focal points, or screen off a private haven such as a woodland area or a wildlife garden.

The way you use trees and hedges in the garden can be tailored to fit your lifestyle. Most trees and shrubs tend to be low-maintenance and offer great garden value for gardeners who are pressed for time. Unlike flowers, with their limited blooming periods, trees and shrubs tend to remain impactful from the depths of winter through to the height of summer.

FOCAL POINTS

Certain trees, such as hawthorns, holly, pears, and some *Sorbus* species, lend themselves especially well to being lightly shaped as they tend to have an intrinsically neat outline and a natural habit that is not too wayward or untidy-looking. They would be useful to punctuate the corners of a square lawn, or to flank a gateway. To endow them with extra impact, plant them in large containers with no bases so they look bigger and more imposing, or plant a distinct low plinth of clipped evergreen plants around their base and/or put an interestingly shaped mowing margin around their trunks.

As you clip the trees in your garden, try experimenting with multistemmed shapes or pyramids, mushrooms, mopheads, or any of the other shapes shown at right.

The quince tree (*Cydonia oblonga*) has a charismatic shape that can be pruned to accentuate its quirkiness. It is fast and easy to grow.

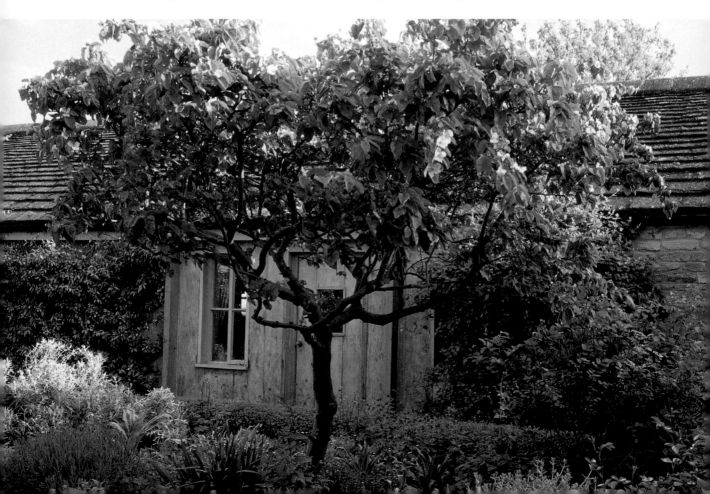

Eight Ways to Emphasize Trees

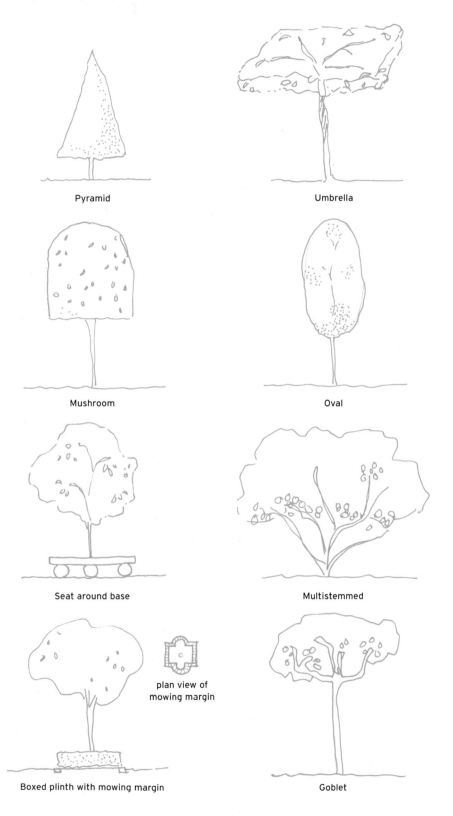

Rather than letting all your trees grow naturally, they can be lightly shaped, tightly clipped, elaborately trained, or emphasized with a seat or basal plinth of planting. Even quite common deciduous trees that you would otherwise not notice will become year-round stunners if they are well sited and given 'the treatment'.

Pyramid

Umbrella

Mushroom

Oval

Seat around base

Multistemmed

plan view of mowing margin

Boxed plinth with mowing margin

Goblet

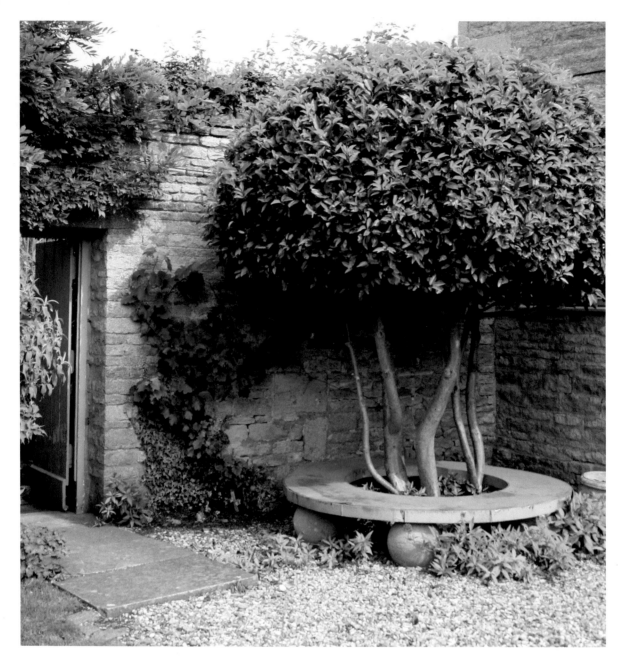

When trees are heavily cut back they respond by growing more quickly—so if you have a tree that is growing weakly on one side, you should cut that weaker-growing side more heavily to encourage it to grow A heavy annual clip encourages a tree to grow vigorously, while a light shape-up does not—so if you only carry out a light clipping every year or so, your tree should still look in good shape. Highly clipped options like pleached trees, however, will become shaggy if they miss out on their regular annual or twice-yearly cutting.

The level of ongoing maintenance that you want to live with will influence your design choices; the more dramatic effects, such as a pleached shape, will work well if you want to carry out a heavy prune once or twice yearly, while the more natural shapes will suit gardeners who foresee carrying out less frequent light pruning sessions.

Foliage has been removed from the lower levels of this Portuguese laurel (*Prunus lusitanica*) to create a small multistemmed focal point.

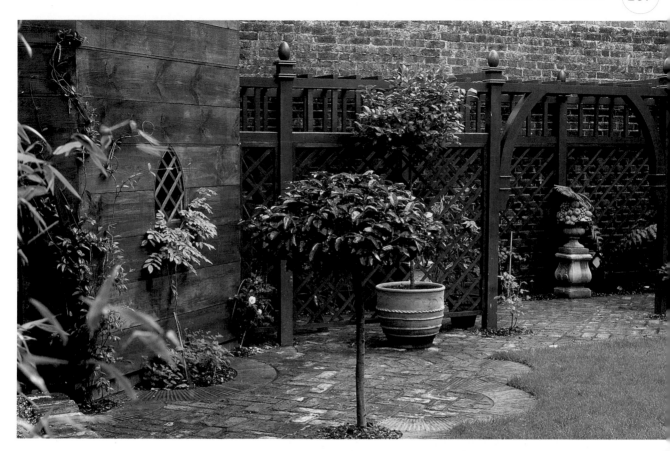

If more permanent, formal outlines suit your preferences and the overall style of your garden, it makes sense to choose evergreen trees, such as the sweet bay (*Laurus nobilis*), the photinia (*Photinia ×fraseri*), the olive (*Olea europaea*) and the fast-growing, wind-resistant evergreen oak (*Quercus ilex*).

When it comes to selecting deciduous trees to shape into focal points, you can choose from a wider spectrum of options. *Platanus*, *Morus* and *Carpinus* species are deservedly popular, and species of *Amelanchier*, *Cornus*, *Sophora*, *Cercis*, some magnolias, and most of the evergreens can be sculpted into superb multistemmed focal points.

If you are impatient, it is possible to buy ready-formed, shapely specimens. However, these have a tendency to be rather expensive and they require a great deal of post-planting care such as watering for a year or more. Forming your own is not as difficult as it may seem; it is highly satisfying, and far less expensive.

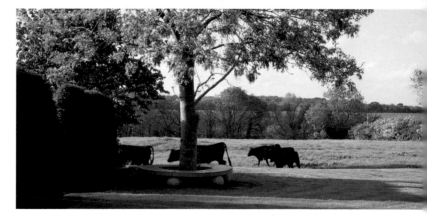

TOP: This recently planted Portuguese laurel is one of four growing at each corner of a small, rectangular lawn. The mowing edge around its base is intricately shaped to add interest. The curved format is made of roofing tiles placed on end.

ABOVE: This ash tree (*Fraxinus excelsior*) sits at the top of an invisible sunken fence. Its lower limbs are regularly removed with a small handsaw to stop the tree from blocking out the view. This also allows the light to reach the grass and adjacent yew hedge below the canopy. Tree work such as this is far easier, and inflicts less shock on the tree, if it is tackled before the limbs become too large.

Designing with Trees and Hedges

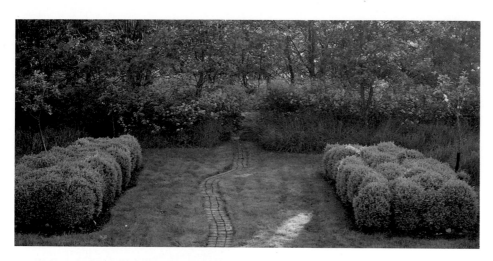

Hedges as Focal Points

Hedges tend to be highly amenable to being sculpted, and when used as focal points they can add a great deal of interest to the garden. Hedges can ape the look of a range of different architectural features such as a series of arches or colonnades. You can even cut windows through dense hedging to showcase tantalizing views.

These can work on a miniature scale; one clipped arch can make a small, otherwise ordinary garden look extraordinarily striking. Also, the most malleable hedges such as *Buxus sempervirens* can be sculpted into dramatic, and even artistic, focal points.

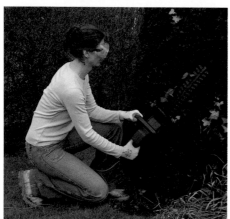

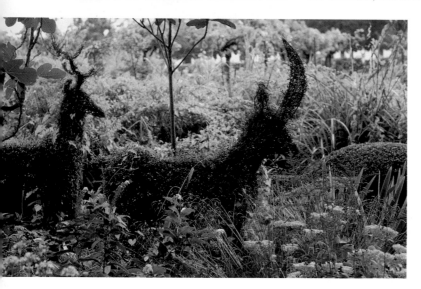

TOP: **These embryonic cloud-pruned hedges define the boundary between mown grass and a wild meadow. They give year-round structure to an otherwise simple space, and require little work beyond an annual clip.**

ABOVE LEFT: **Goggles and gloves should be worn when using a power-assisted hedge trimmer. Try to situate yourself side-on to the hedge, bending your knees to give yourself a stable base. Keep your shoulder blades relaxed, not hunched.**

LEFT: **Hedges offer ample scope for fun and creativity!**

RIGHT: **Although I am using hand pruners (secateurs) here, I often use mechanical hedge cutters, or single- or double-handed shears. For show gardens, I sometimes even use a regular pair of scissors.**

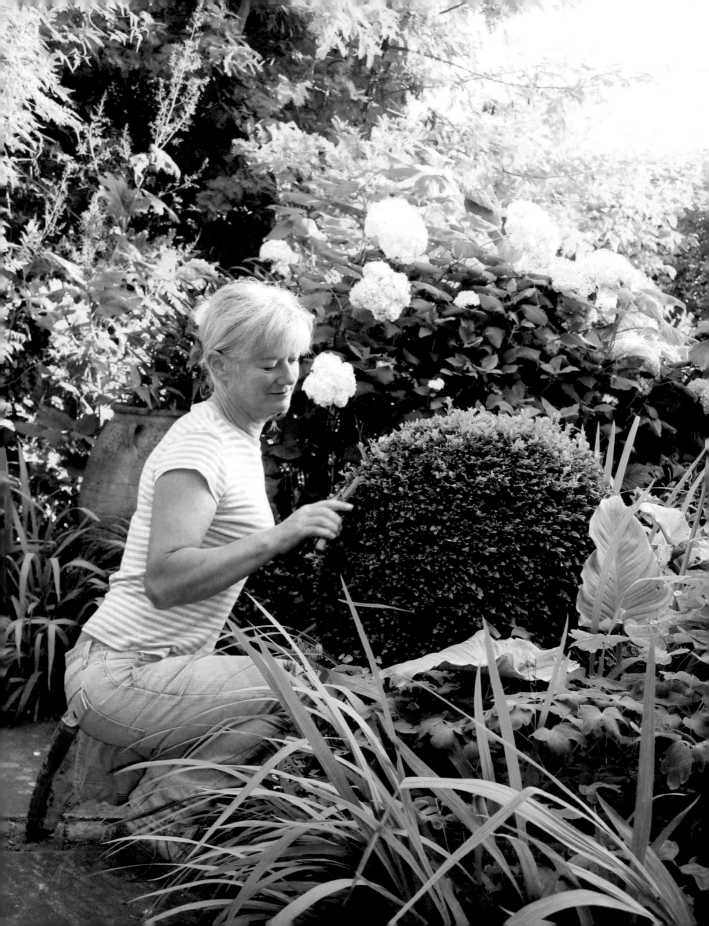

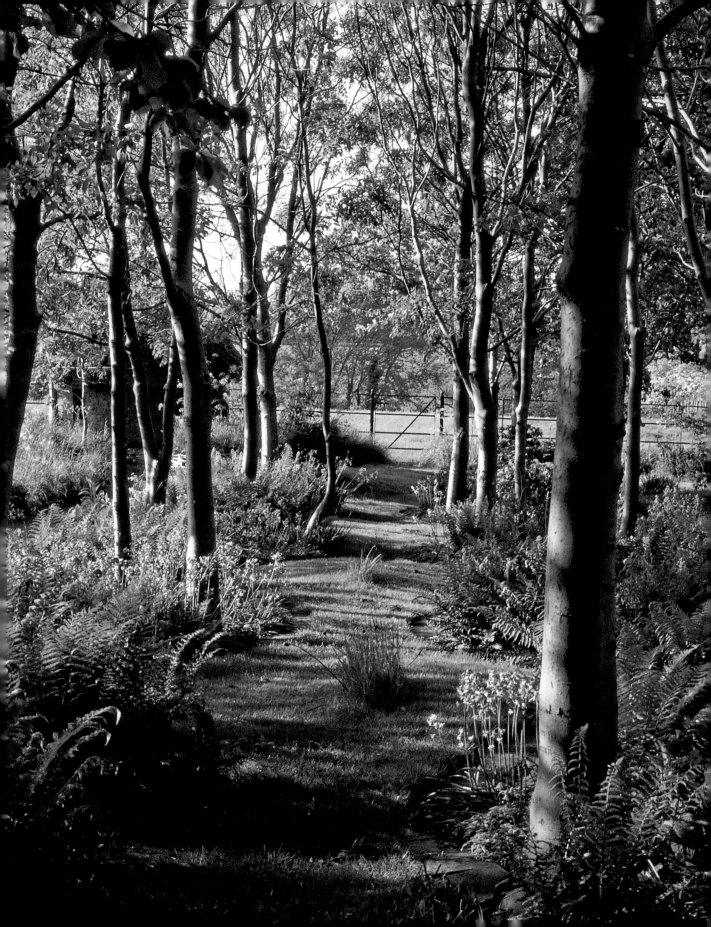

SCREENING AND INTERNAL BOUNDARIES

For some inexplicable reason, it seems that the eye is always immediately drawn to the ugliest feature in the garden, which can take attention away from its more attractive elements. Trees and hedges offer the opportunity to personalize your garden, framing your favourite views and screening out less desirable ones. An avenue of quince trees might emphasize your front door, while a line of pleached hornbeam can ably shield the sight of your neighbour's caravan from your driveway. A tunnel of fruit trees can frame the path to your greenhouse, or a colonnade of box hedging can highlight a stunning view across the fields. Crucially, taller trees and hedges can also be strategically placed to maximize privacy. They can shield outdoor spaces from being overlooked by neighbours or glimpsed from the road, creating a private haven for relaxation, strolling, or—perhaps most importantly—exercising.

In larger gardens particularly, the space can sometimes seem very sprawling and open, which can make it feel somehow less than welcoming, as well as—surprisingly—smaller. Trees and shrubs can give your space the feeling of being enclosed and work like an outdoor room. They also provide shelter from battering winds and storms, and filter out smoke, fumes and environmental pollution and reduce noise, creating a microclimate that is hospitable to wildlife as well as human beings.

For most of us, practising Pilates in a private, screened-out woodland floor beats doing so in a crowded gym. You might add a simplified trim trail with a basic bench designed for a range of exercises, a few stretching posts, and a perhaps a small balancing rail that will encourage you to warm up before gardening, work your muscles, and stretch out afterwards.

Using trees and hedges to form spaces and focus viewpoints can add tremendous impact to a garden and make it highly individual without requiring large amounts of maintenance (although the designing and planting require foresight). It is important to keep all grass and weed competition well away from them; without competition from grasses, trees and hedges grow about 60% more quickly.

Using Trees for Screening

A tree screen can take many different forms. Because a screen can be quite dominant, it sometimes makes sense to complement a functional screen with one or more additional 'screens'. Even if these extra screens are not actually screening anything out, they can serve to balance the design and possibly help direct the viewpoint in a totally new direction. This has the effect of disguising the purpose of the screen planting, making it far more effective (see photo on page 163).

Sometimes space is limited and the plants need to have their canopies trained and confined so they will grow near to buildings without causing structural damage or blocking out too much light. It is not always necessary to have a solid screen to hide an adjacent building; sometimes, just breaking up a dominant roofline is enough to hide the worst sections. Similarly, the height of the eventual screen may not need to go to the top of building or object; instead, it might just hide the highest row of windows.

Do not assume that it is essential for your screen to be completely evergreen. Deciduous trees tend to grow faster and in winter a dense framework of twigs hides a substantial amount. Try looking through a dense hawthorn hedge in winter—you can see precious little, especially when viewed from an angle.

When planning your screen, always try to imagine how the space will look once everything is fully grown and mature. It helps to put up strings at different heights, in order to get a sense of the height to which you need the trees to grow to minimize the effect of the eyesore.

Apart from conifers, evergreen trees are often slow growing—so unless you import large, formed trees such as evergreen oaks, photinias, bay, or laurel, they require patience. Deciduous trees make good screens as they are faster growing. If you have space, consider planting a line of fast-growing deciduous trees with a line of young, evergreen trees beside them. As soon as the evergreens reach the desired proportions, remove the faster screen plants. The illustrations on the following page show a range of different options for making ornamental and useful screens.

LEFT: These trees were planted from tiny transplants about twenty years ago. Young whips are fast to establish, need no staking, and form a better shape than larger ones. The low-maintenance ground cover includes ferns, bluebells, foxgloves, and a few wildflowers.

Designing with Trees and Hedges

Line

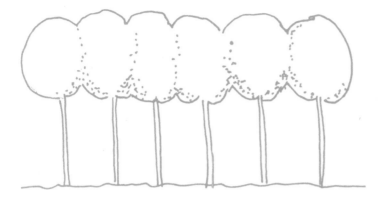

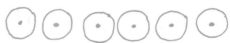

When planting trees in a simple line, you should choose deciduous trees that retain their leaves for a long time if you want a quick screen. One example is the medium-sized *Pyrus calleryana* 'Chanticleer' which has glossy, long-lasting leaves that form a dense canopy. It has a narrow head, is vigorous and could be planted at 6 ft. (2 m) centres to form a neat, strong line. Prune gently to maintain a shapely effect.

Allée

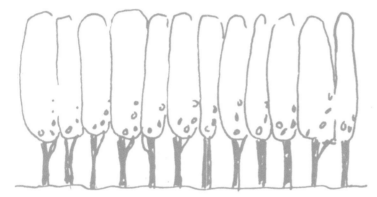

PLAN

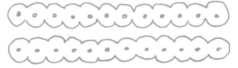

An allée consist of a double line of trees, usually planted close together so they can be used in small-scale gardens and to line quite narrow paths. The trees in each line may be just 2 ft. (60 cm) apart so that they form a wall of foliage. To keep the form strong and bold, the point where the trees' trunks ends and their canopies begin should be uniform, as should the height of the treetops—so it helps to use just one type of tree. For a formal, tall, and dense look, clipped evergreen oak is ideal; hazel, contrastingly, would be less formal, and fairly transparent in winter. Pear, beech, hornbeam, lime, birch, sorbus, and yew trees would all work nicely.

Bottomless Containers

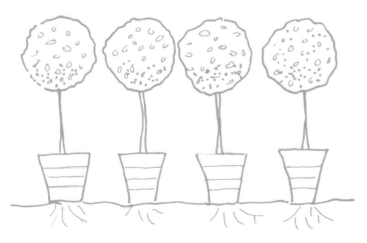

PLAN

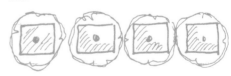

This is a quick method for creating eye-level screens. Use large containers (at least 2 ft., or 60 cm, high and wide), with no bases so that the plants are able to root into the soil below. After a year, no watering is usually necessary and the roots' anchorage stops them from blowing over.

Pleached

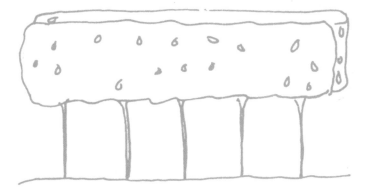

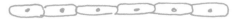

Here trees are planted between 5 ft. (1.5 m) and 9 ft. 8 in. (3 m) apart. You then train them by taking a lateral branch that is tied onto a horizontal bamboo cane or wire and joining it up with a corresponding lateral branch on the adjacent tree. The result is a series of between four and twelve horizontal tiers of connected branches. The laterals that grow away from this plane of growth are cut off, so that you see only what is effectively a hedge of foliage that is about 1-2 yards (or metres) off the ground. The effect is highly architectural, and because you have relatively open space at base of the trees it allows you to create walkways, borders, and paths underneath them. This adds a sense of depth which is very valuable in a confined garden.

Tunnels

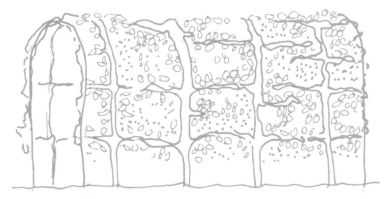

PLAN

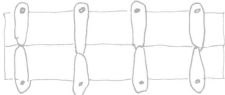

A natural progression from an allée is a tunnel of trees to screen up to a height of 6.5-9 ft. (2-3 m) or more. Hornbeam, beech, hawthorn, and other smaller-leaved trees will form a dense mass of green that can be cut with hedge clippers. Apples, pears, and willows make fabulous tunnels but they do not form such dense structures. Metal arches can provide the framework and the trees can be planted at close centres (19-in. or 50-cm).

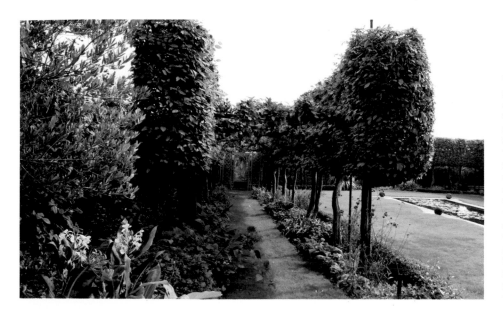

This double line of pleached hornbeam (*Carpinus betulus*) was planted to screen an ugly, overlooking building on one side. The presence of the screen on both sides of the pool takes attention away from the eyesore. These trees were planted as 1-ft. (30-cm) high transplants and after about eight years they had much impact as a result of pruning that directed the growth where it was needed.

Designing with Trees and Hedges

Using Hedges for Internal Boundaries

Unless your garden is tiny, creating boundaries with hedging will make it more liveable and user-friendly as you delineate areas you can use for relaxing, strolling, playing and of course indulging in some exercise. Even a hedge that is below eye level will define a separate space. Hedging is generally a low-maintenance option, so if you like your garden to look structured and interesting throughout the year, and you have not much time to cultivate and tend borders, then this is an important section for you.

Hedges need not be in long, straight, unbroken lines. Curvaceous, snaking serpentine hedges look dynamic and modern, although the serpentine is a classical shape and so fits in well with period buildings too.

Regular straight blocks with gaps between have an interesting rhythm about them and entice you to look at the spaces between. A hedge that has regular buttresses along its length takes on an architectural feel; in this situation the buttresses are not for extra stability, as on a masonry wall. Instead, they

TRICKLE IRRIGATION

If you can apply a trickle irrigation pipe along the length of the hedge that drips out water around the base of the plant in dry, hot weather, you will speed up your hedge's growth enormously. Even yew hedging, which hates winter wet, will grow far more quickly if it is watered in dry periods. In fact, with copious water in the summer, yew hedging can put on staggering growth rates.

When your hedge has reached the desired height, you can slowly wean it off the irrigation, encouraging it to develop deeper roots, so that its new growth does not become excessive and difficult to maintain.

are there to embellish and add extra depth and texture. Combining greenery with bricks and mortar is a good way to make hedges look more architectural. You can add brick or stone piers to the ends, put gates or doorways through them or build a low plinth wall along the front so that the hedge eventually grows 'on' it.

These yew panels were grown from cuttings. Only the sides (not the tops) were cut until the panels grew to 1 ft. (30 cm) from the desired height.

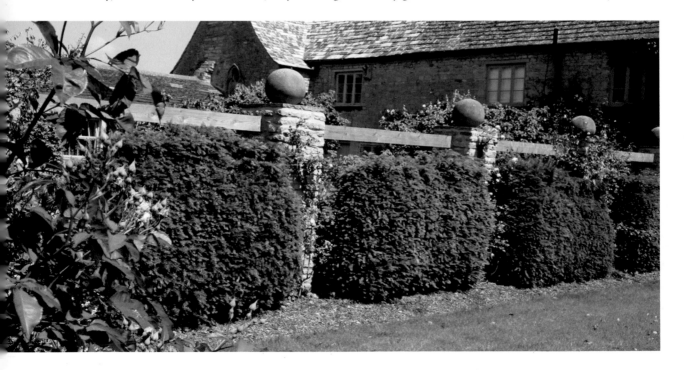

Sawing

Old trees can look stately, but they need to be checked regularly as their falling limbs could endanger people or buildings. If you have trees overhanging paths, roads, or buildings, you need to be extra-vigilant about checking them for signs of ill health. Keep in mind that if you have disturbed the soil under the canopy this can jeopardize the tree's health.

Make a habit of scrutinizing them on a regular basis as you walk around the garden. Call in a professionally qualified arborist if you notice fungi, limbs that appear dead, excessively long or heavy, large cracks and cavities in the tree, or a generally decrepit appearance.

If you choose to remove young branches on your own, you can take steps to protect yourself from injury. To make the job easier, it is best to stand sideways onto the tree and hold onto a sturdy branch with one hand as you saw.

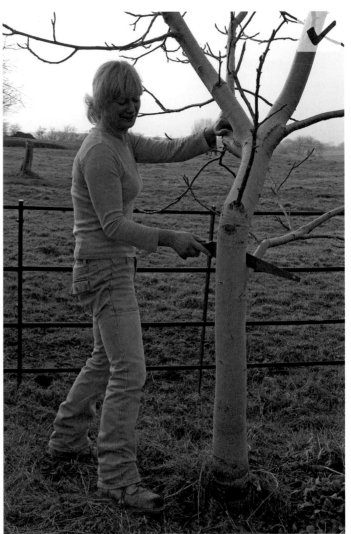

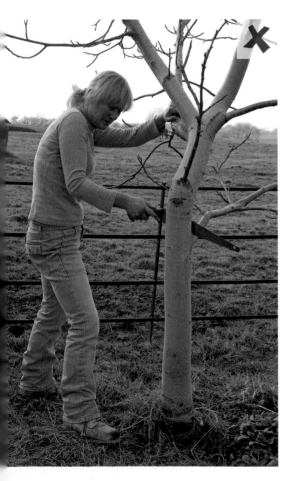

LEFT: **Sawing like this places undue stress on your neck and shoulders.**

ABOVE: **As you move the saw back and forth, keep it as level as possible and transfer your weight between your front and back feet with each motion. Keep your lower abdominals lifted to minimize any stress this might place on your spine. Make sure that your shoulders remain relaxed, with your shoulder blades pressed down into the centre of your upper back.**

Low-Maintenance Wildlife Gardens

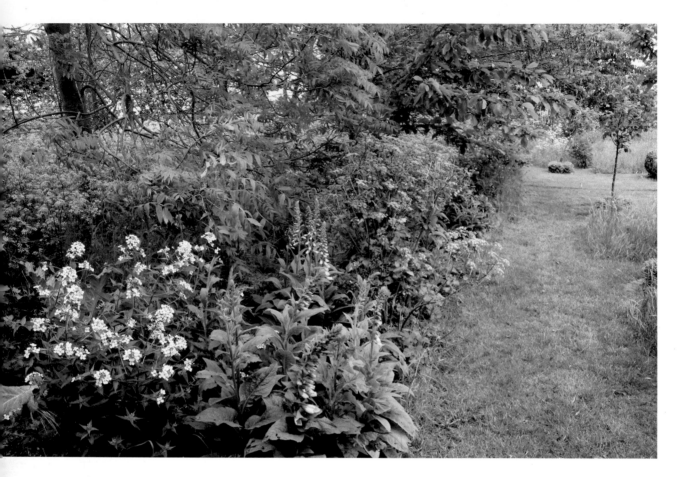

Cultivating appealing spaces that attract wildlife gives a fresh dimension to gardens, bringing outdoor spaces to life and effecting a vivid connection to nature that tends to enhance overall wellbeing. In a garden designed to invite wildlife you can watch birds build their nests and listen to the melodic sounds of bees buzzing around foxgloves and birds singing. With simple planning, you can create areas that attract populations of owls, nuthatches, greater spotted woodpeckers and many small mammals and insects.

To boost the wildlife population in your garden, provide as many different types of habitat as you can: native shrubby areas, a native tree or two, some wildflowers, and a mown glade. Bird feeders will also be a boon to the space. If you enjoy fish, frogs,

newts, and other water-dwelling creatures, consider adding a body of water such as a pond or a naturalistic pool, which will bring a hugely interesting dimension. This can require a little work, yet it is frequently magnetic (to wildlife and gardeners alike).

MAINTAINING A HEALTHY BALANCE

With their longer grass, wildflowers, and variety of habitats, wildlife gardens may appear relaxed. Yet maintaining a variety of different habitats that coexist in harmony requires that you keep a careful eye on the plants. In areas where grass, flowers, trees, and shrubs have been allowed to grow a bit more freely, some plants—particularly the perennial invasive ones—can become too established and dominant.

This easygoing border includes a mix of foxgloves, sweet rocket, cowslips, and other wildflowers. In the evenings it attracts bats that swoop over the border in pursuit of insects.

Nettles (*Urtica dioica*), for instance, are a mixed blessing. On one hand, they attract wildlife to the garden. Small tortoiseshell, red admiral, and peacock caterpillars live on them, toads and frogs can often be found in their thicker clumps, and aphids gravitate towards them and, in turn, invite ladybirds. They also make fabulous compost material, and their young leaves can be a tasty and wholesome addition to soup. However, in meadows they can become too much of a good thing, especially when they seed around prolifically into nearby borders. Their yellow, wiry roots are not that deep-growing, and on wet days after heavy rain it is satisfying to pull them out, leaves, shoots, roots, and all—but make sure you wear gauntlets. The best solution may be to keep some clumps of nettles in the backwaters of your garden.

Although they require some work, areas designed to attract wildlife carry a major advantage—they essentially make life easier and less stressful in the garden. When you decide to abandon the ideal of an entirely manicured, neat, and sterile look, you become free to choose the most convenient and enjoyable time to do things. If you are

extremely busy, you can delay jobs to suit your preferences, so that if you do not have time to thin the aquatic vegetation from the pool one month, you can do it the next, and if you forget to mow the grass path one week, it will not appear out of place and overly shaggy the following week.

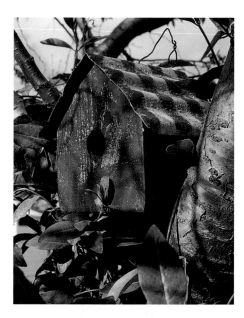

BELOW LEFT: **When we tidy up our gardens by removing dead trees, brambles, and other wilder spaces, birds are left with fewer nesting spaces. Adding a simple bird box helps to compensate for this.**

BELOW: **It is well known that butterflies are magnetically attracted to buddlejas. Adding a range of different buddleja species will bring attractive splashes of colour (as well as welcome butterflies) to the wildlife garden.**

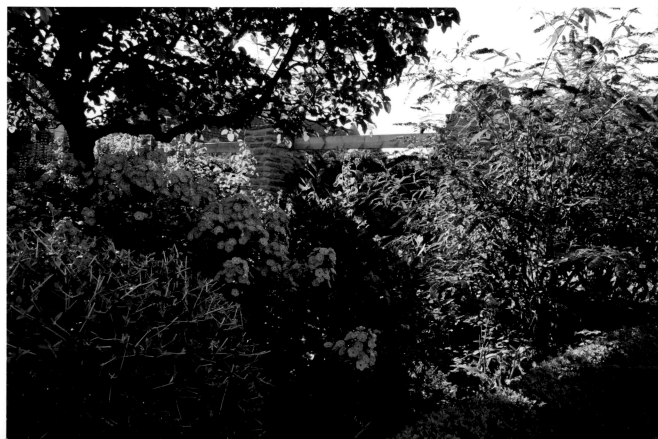

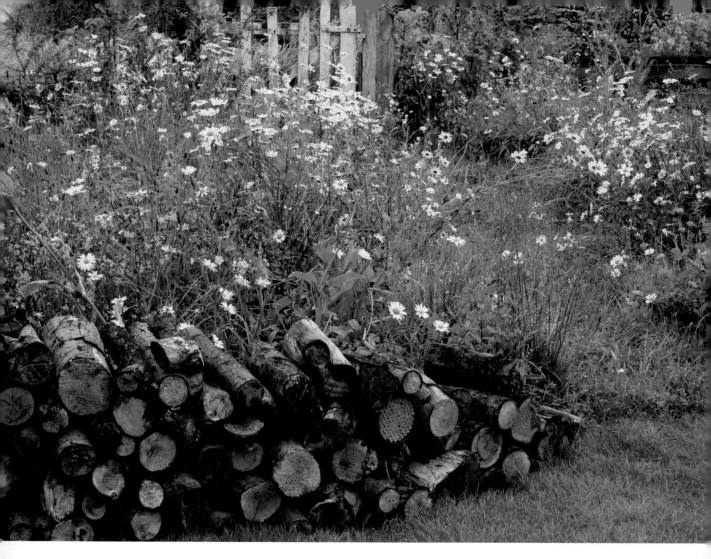

Of course, an overly lax approach to garden maintenance tasks can backfire: if you let things go for too long, you may attack jobs more spasmodically so that when you finally get around to trimming your wildflower meadow you will spend hours using muscles which have not been extended for weeks or months. Try to protect yourself by spreading the maintenance burden over a longer period, doing a bit each weekend or an odd evening every so often. Warm your body up first, and stretch afterwards—and if your muscles start to twinge or grumble mid-task, remember to take a break.

Wildlife gardens are all about balance. You want to attract as much wildlife in as you can but you do not want a wilderness so you offend your neighbours and make your house look derelict. If the pernicious weeds become out of hand and you end up with monocultures of Japanese knotweed and mare's tails, then the people next door will have a problem (plus, you will not be attracting a rich range of butterflies and birds). It is fantastic having decaying wood, rotting leaves and other matter for fungi and invertebrates to colonize, but instead of leaving them where they fall in highly visible places, collect them up and spread them under hedge bottoms or in piles in woodland or under trees. Here they will form a weed-suppressing mulch and help to reduce evaporation.

Certain sections of the garden, such as the entrance area and driveway, can still give a more structured and cultivated impression, even though it is a wildlife garden. You may want to boost the more muted colours of some native thicket planting by adding wallflowers in spring, followed by forget-me-nots and tobacco plants. You may also

This log wall takes very little time to build and is highly worthwhile as it provides great cracks and crevices for small animals to hide in.

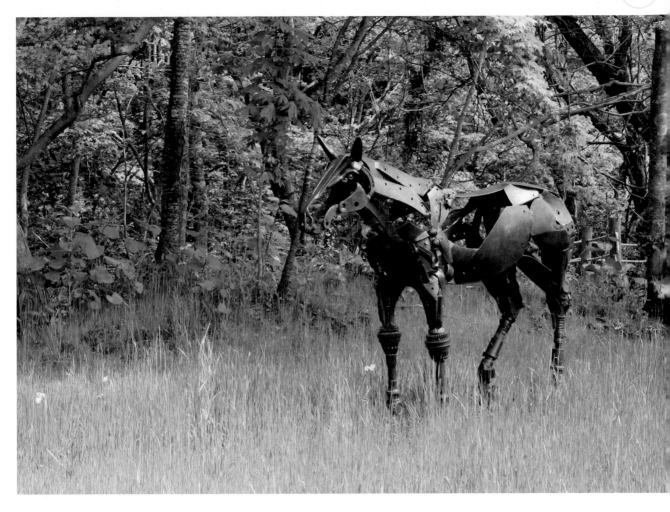

wish to inject some exotic bulbs such as camassias and species tulips into your sheets of native daffodils in the meadow.

As you perform maintenance tasks such as weeding, try to create as little disturbance to the inhabitants as possible. This is one environment where you should try to avoid introducing fertilizers or chemicals; instead, look for alternative ways to tackle challenges. If your roses are continually being attacked by black spot and mildew, try to use more disease-resistant species, do not group them all together, introduce mycorrhizae on planting them so they are not as stressed, mulch them well to conserve moisture, and jettison those that are not 'happy'.

Because of the variability of the changing seasons and the unpredictable nature of pests and diseases, gardeners encounter many problems as they grow and change.

If your garden looks like a million dollars just once in a rare while, that may suit you well. Alternatively, rather than striving for flawlessness, it can be far more satisfying to achieve a well-balanced and life-enhancing space that you and the wildlife can enjoy. During seasons when the wildlife-attracting areas are lacking in colour and flowers, adding sculpture gives impact to the space.

Perhaps the most attractive thing about low-maintenance planting schemes is that they afford you more time to relax and simply appreciate your space. With the time you would otherwise spend striving to achieve an emerald-striped lawn or a dizzyingly intricate flower border, you can do some regular deep breathing exercises as you wander around feeding visiting birds, or practise body-balancing Pilates next to a sweet-smelling, flourishing, and cleverly designed flower border.

This horse sculpture, created by Helen Denerley, is made entirely from scrap metal objects. It 'lives' in the Ginga Garden, Japan.

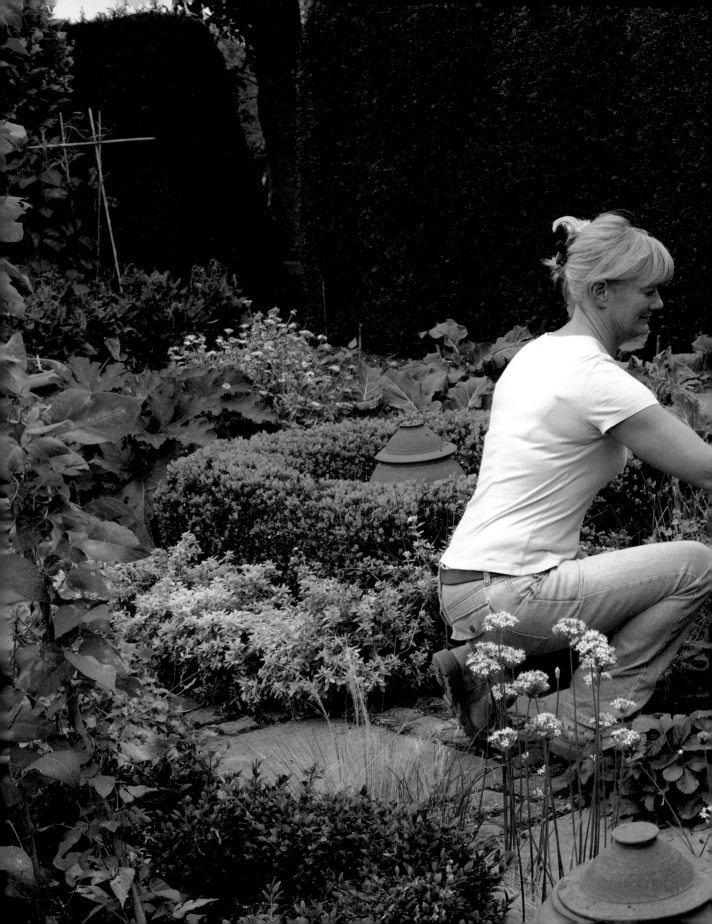

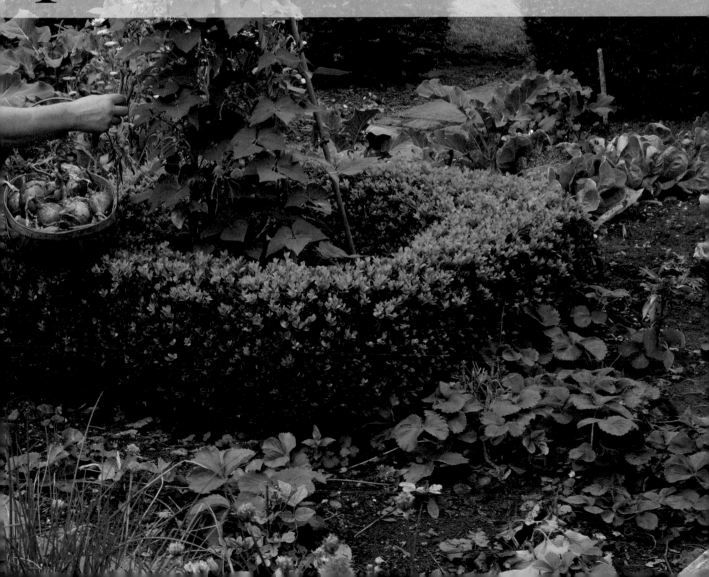

health and fitness in
THE PRODUCTIVE GARDEN

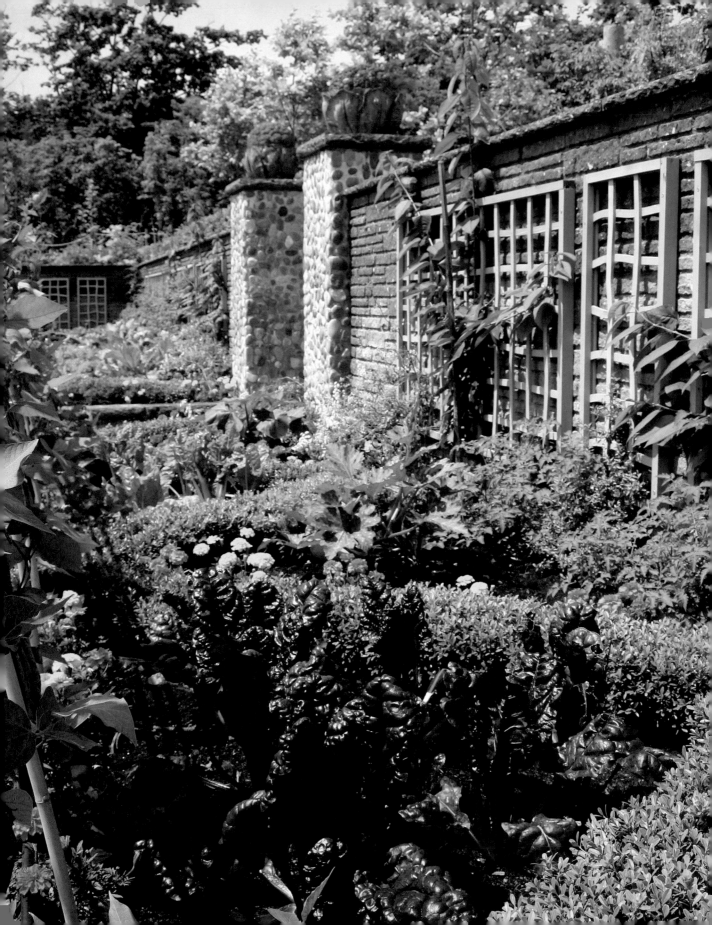

CULTIVATING FRUITS, vegetables, nuts, and herbs is one of the most healthy and satisfying things we can do in our gardens. It was once thought to be hard and frustrating work, requiring a serious investment of time, expansive space, and strenuous graft. But in recent years productive gardens have boomed in popularity across North America, Great Britain, and elsewhere, and in the process gardeners have been awakening to a wealth of techniques that can save time, reduce frustration, and make a garden brimming with healthy produce an altogether more attainable ideal.

Growing your own produce can be as easy or as challenging as you want it to be. A constantly evolving edible garden will keep you focused and active, urging you to limber up and work out on a regular basis as you bend to sow seeds, move around to weed beds, and stretch skyward to pick fruit in the fresh air. If your workspace—comprising, for instance, a compost heap, potting bench, and storage shed—is designed to fit your needs, this will also reduce frustration and make your experience more rewarding. Regardless of how much time you are able to spend maintaining your garden, it pays to choose plants that are consistently good performers and require less effort. These include the perennial vegetables, reliable fruit and nut trees, and health-enhancing herbs highlighted throughout this chapter, most of which are capable of yielding wonderfully nutritious produce with little upkeep.

Edible gardens may have been banished to out-of-the-way places in the past, but they can look extremely inviting if you design their growing space to fit a matrix or patternwork of small beds. You can then position them in full view, in a convenient spot near the kitchen so that a last-minute dash outside for a fresh herb to enhance a salad is not a chore, but rather a pleasure.

In the Ginga Gardens in Hokkaido, Japan, raised vegetable beds have been divided into smaller triangular shapes surrounded by low box hedging. Each area is home to a single vegetable type; the purple chard in the foreground is easy to grow.

Why Grow Your Own?

The hours spent growing and preparing food may have been considered laborious by our ancestors, but now that fast food and processed snacks are ubiquitous, taking the time to produce and prepare our own food becomes something of a luxury. Growing and cooking different seasonal crops throughout the year helps bring variation and excitement to our diets, and offers an alternative to the predictable, processed, and often imported food that we have grown accustomed to buying in stores. It is always satisfying to dig up the first crop of new potatoes that you have nurtured along in your sunniest spot, especially as they have a taste far superior to those all-year-round, packaged imports. Perhaps most importantly, growing your own food and eating it when freshly picked is often the healthiest option of all.

NUTRITIONAL VALUE AND TASTINESS

When it comes to nutritional value, the food you grow in your own garden will invariably be superior to the produce available on supermarkets' shelves. Commercially grown vegetables are selected for their good shelf life, uniform cropping, colour, high yield, and sometimes for their large size; flavour and nutrient content tend to rank lower on supermarkets' list of priorities, and while your homegrown fruits and vegetables may not look as large or as perfect as those grown commercially, they will probably taste much better. Their nutritional value will be especially high if you eat them soon after picking.

In many vegetables, certain changes take place that diminish flavour soon after picking. One of the easiest to detect is the conversion of sugars to starch. In peas and sweetcorn, this is especially noticeable—freshly picked sweetcorn and peas taste incredibly sweet, but if you wait even a few hours the quality of that taste declines. This is because the sugars begin to change into starch the moment these vegetables are picked. Nutrient loss, too, is inevitable when fruits and vegetables are stored over time.

A 2004 study on bagged spinach showed that after picking, the spinach leaves lost a substantial amount of nutrients as they were kept at various storage temperatures, and it is probable that bagged salads experience similar nutrient loss. Broccoli has also been shown to lose nutrients quickly; in an experiment at the University of Warwick in England, it was shown that the Vitamin C content of broccoli had fallen by about 50% four days after it was picked. Other studies have suggested that many other fruits and vegetables lose nutrients at a similar rate, so growing them yourself and eating them soon after picking will ensure that you get optimum nutritional value.

GOING ORGANIC

For gardeners who are both health-conscious and environmentally aware, going organic is often an especially attractive option in the edible garden. Although there is conflicting evidence on whether organic food is healthier, research has strongly suggested that organically grown produce may contain significantly more Vitamin C, iron, magnesium, and phosphorous and a lower nitrate content than inorganic crops.

You also can endeavour to keep the soil in good condition so that the nutrient content of your vegetables is as high as possible. You can do this by using organic manures and compost in preference to encouraging lots of soft, rapid growth by pumping them with water and inorganic fertilizers. It also helps to choose varieties of vegetables and fruits that have been shown to grow well under organic conditions. These varieties may have more extensive root systems to utilize nutrients, they may be selected for vigorous leaf growth to compete with weedier conditions and they may be less vulnerable to diseases. (Be prepared to tolerate a bit of slug and aphid damage, and also to rinse your produce well in salted water before cooking—otherwise, you might encounter a bit of unexpected protein on your plate.)

Bear in mind that although a totally organic productive garden may be appealing, it is also important to be

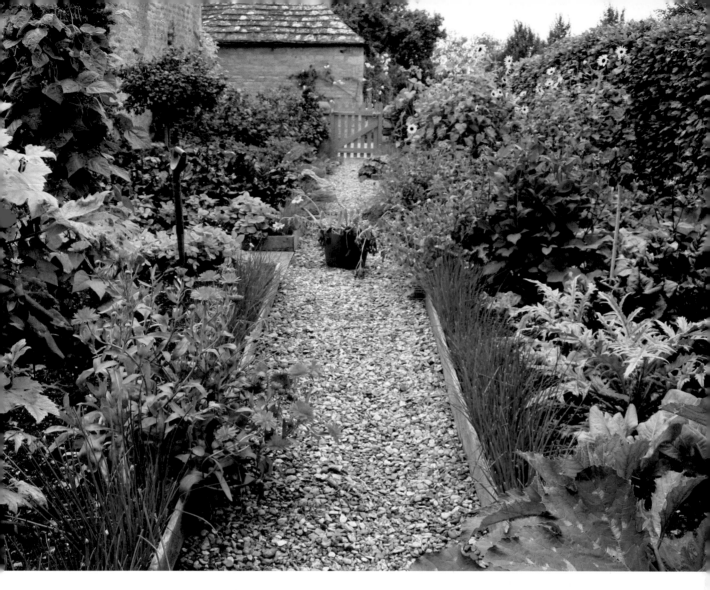

Marigolds and sunflowers add splashes of colour to a highly productive space.

pragmatic. If your garden experiences a massive attack by one particular pest one year, resorting to an inorganic chemical may be the best way to avoid giving up or losing the afflicted crop. Even if you need to occasionally resort to chemicals in the productive garden, the food you grow is likely to be better in many ways than the store-bought alternative. You may even find that you eat more vegetables, as they will taste so delicious.

ENVIRONMENTAL RESPONSIBILITY

As global warming and carbon dioxide emissions become increasingly concerning, we are all becoming more aware of the impact of air miles. When it comes to eschewing food that has travelled around

the world in favour of locally sourced produce, even small decisions can make an important impact. For instance, when the ethical farming group SUSTAIN analyzed a sample basket of imported organic vegetables, they found that they had travelled a distance equivalent to six times around the equator—a trip that will have released as much carbon dioxide into the atmosphere as a four-bedroom household cooking meals over eight months. SUSTAIN also discovered that locally grown spring onions bought through a box scheme in Britain would generate three hundred times less carbon dioxide than a bunch flown in from Mexico. If you are able to pick a few fresh leaves or pods of peas right on your doorstep with zero air miles, then this is something in which to take immense pride.

Working in the Edible Garden

When you work in the garden, you often feel as though there is a small part of you in it, rather like a child that you tend and shape. Both can be unpredictable, throwing up unexpected surprises (both good and bad), and this unpredictability can motivate you to stay active as you monitor the progress of a succulent new variety of baby fennel or check whether your globe artichokes will be plump enough to harvest.

Fruits and vegetables benefit from sustained, regular attention. This does not necessarily mean lots of hard work; much of it involves keeping an eye out for slug activity, evaluating when you need to pinch out the tops of beans, or checking to see whether your sweetcorn is ripe for the picking. If you can incorporate a series of exercises into your regular strolls around the kitchen garden, so much the better.

These days, many gardeners have been choosing to sow fewer seeds in the open ground and more in modular trays that are kept in a protected space like a greenhouse, a cold frame, or a sheltered corner. This way, the seeds become tough, small plants before they have to cope with slugs, pests, downpours, early frosts, and other adverse conditions; as weather conditions become more and more unpredictable, this often makes a great deal of sense. (If you want to sidestep sowing your own seeds, many companies will sell small plug plants to fill the gap; make sure that you harden them off for a week of two before planting them in their final position.)

SUCCESSFUL SEED SOWING

These measures will increase your chance of success when sowing in containers.
• Do not use ordinary garden soil; instead, use a sowing and potting compost for seed trays.
• Moisten the compost prior to sowing by immersing the tray in water, then firm well when drained.
• All but the smallest seeds should be covered with a thin layer of compost or fine-grade vermiculite to a depth of ¼ in. (6 mm). (If the seeds are particularly large,

you can use ½ in. (12 mm) of fine-grade vermiculite.) This will keep seeds warm while keeping in moisture and preventing algal growth on the surface.
• Covering seeds with clingfilm will prevent them from drying out quickly (but watch out for mould).
• To speed up germination, seeds can be left in a warm, dark place (near to a radiator, for instance) and then moved back to the light immediately after they germinate.
• Peas, French (green) beans, and runner (string) beans can be placed on moist kitchen towel initially, and then planted either in situ or in modules as soon as they begin to swell up or chit. (Do not damage the embryonic shoot or root.)
• Never plant out seedlings until they have been hardened off for a week or two, as their leaf structure will be vulnerable to pests, disease, and inclement weather.
• Water seeds from below until they look quite sturdy, or use a watering can with a fine rose.

HINTS FOR SHADY AREAS OR INFERTILE SOIL

To maximize your chances of cultivating a rewarding productive garden, it is obviously best to avoid planting in areas with notorious 'problem conditions' such as shade or infertile soil. However, if you have no choice, you can take certain measures to counteract the challenging conditions.

If the soil is waterlogged or dry and thin, aim to correct this before you start, creating raised beds or adding volumes of organic compost can boost most soils to productive levels. Although shade can be a restricting factor in city gardens, you can help to alleviate it by raising beds up, or thinning or raising the adjacent canopies of trees. Painting adjacent walls or fences in light colours to reflect the sunlight can make a substantial difference, too. Some vegetables cope better with shade than others: Jerusalem artichokes, Chinese cabbage, gooseberries, Chinese chives, chrysanthemum greens, cucumbers, endives, parsley, peas, mizuna greens, spinach, and sorrel are a few examples. Fruits that can thrive in light shade include gooseberries, raspberries, rhubarbs, and redcurrants.

Digging

Digging in the productive garden is hard work and it makes sense to pause from time to time. Rest, walk around the garden, or carry out a different activity every fifteen minutes. Practising good technique helps your body to remain balanced, lessening your vulnerability to strain and injury.

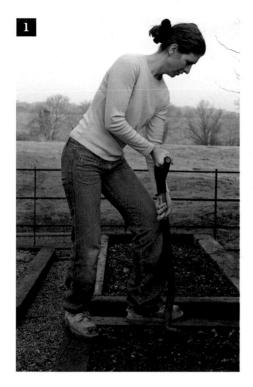

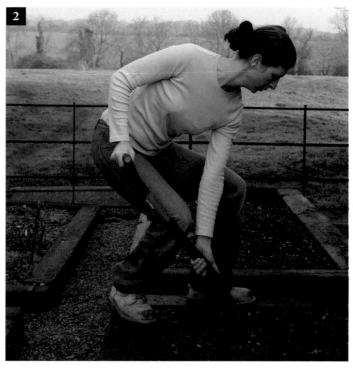

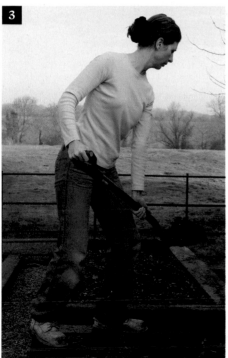

1 Place one foot on the spade and prepare by engaging the deep stabilizing muscles in your lower stomach, lifting these muscles up and in. Leaning slightly forward and keeping your back in neutral, push downward so that the spade sinks into the soil.

2 With your foot still on the spade, lever back on it to loosen the soil if necessary. As your body crouches lower, the movement should stem from your hip rather than your lower back.

3 Take your foot off of the spade. Your arms then take over to shift the soil. Your knees should be slightly bent, with one foot in front of the other, and your lower abdominal muscles should remain lifted up and in. As the soil is lifted up, your stomach muscles and arms take the load. At this point it is a good idea to move your feet to put the soil in place, rather than twisting your back. Try to alternate sides for a more balanced exercise.

Working in the Edible Garden

DETERRING PESTS AND DISEASES

In addition to daily vigilance, a range of measures will help to protect your productive garden, keeping irritants at bay.

Get your soil in great heart with organic mulches; soft growth triggered by a high-nitrogen diet and copious irrigation is more susceptible to many pest and diseases. If you have a big slug problem, use ferric phosphate slug pellets (approved by Garden Organic). These are not only extremely efficient but they also last well in wet conditions. Use fleece and netting to protect crops such as carrots and brassicas, which are vulnerable to pest including carrot fly, cabbage root fly, and cabbage white butterfly. It often helps to grow varieties of plants tipped as great for organic gardening as they tend to be more vigorous and resistant to pests and diseases.

Get to know your beneficial insects. Ladybird larvae feed on aphids, as do larvae of hoverflies and lacewings. Encourage fast-moving bugs such as centipedes that generally feed on plant-eaters such as slugs and slow-moving insects. Frogs and toads also eat slugs, and so are assets to the edible garden.

Grow flowers for nectar and pollen, too; plants with flowers that are small, or flat and open are good for this purpose. Pot marigolds (*Calendula officinalis*), fennel (*Foeniculum vulgare*), and thyme (*Thymus* species) are worthwhile additions to the mix, as they confuse pests and attract their predators. Try interplanting carrots with love-in-a-mist (*Nigella damascena*), blue flax (*Linum usitatissimum*), and scabious (*Knautia arvensis*) within blocks of carrots to confuse and deter the carrot fly. If you are growing broad beans, pinching out the

Dividing your plot into miniature beds makes crops easier to reach and helps with rotation. Each square holds one crop, and even when a square becomes empty the overall layout still looks appealing.

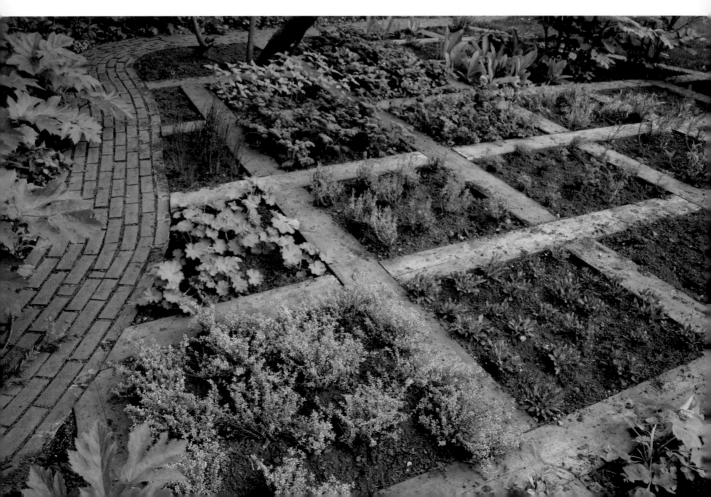

tops once the first pod has set will help to deter black bean aphids. Interplanting in this way will confound pests that prey on a particular species.

Certain annual vegetables are simpler to grow and far less troublesome than others. Climbing French (green) beans are often easier than runner (string) beans, especially in hot summers. Courgettes (zucchini), leeks, garlic, broad (fava) beans, cut-and-come-again lettuces, spinach, beetroot, spring onions (scallions), parsnips, onions, potatoes, and chilli peppers are prone to very few pests and diseases.

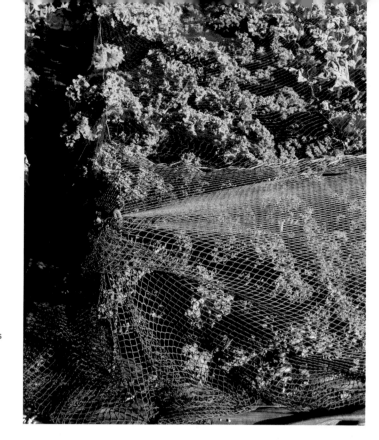

BELOW: In Annie Huntingdon's garden, the vegetables are laid out in real style. Diagonal rows are visually pleasing and the lettuces are grown in pairs so that when one is picked, the other remains to keep up appearances.

RIGHT: Brassicas are delicious, but they are often targeted by pests. Here metal pins are used to support netting which is held just off the crop so that the cabbage white butterflies cannot lay eggs on the leaves.

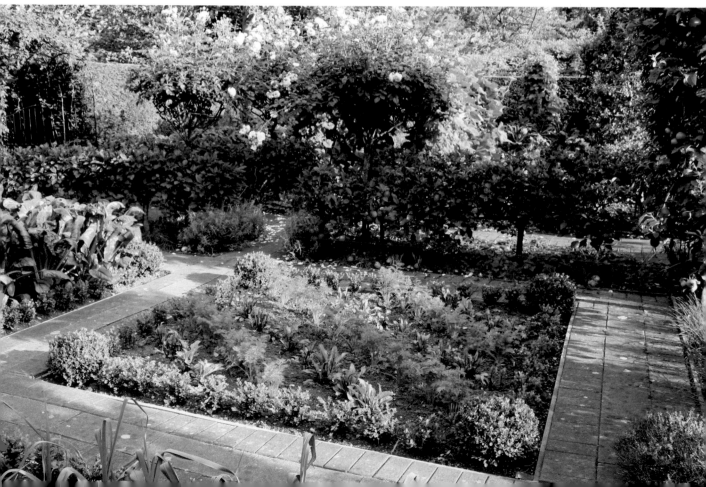

Working in the Edible Garden

MAINTAINING A HEALTHY EDIBLE GARDEN

Once your plants are established, your work in the edible garden may involve using a draw hoe and picking crops that are low to the ground.

It is important to perform these actions in a way that keeps your body balanced, so try to switch sides as much as possible.

Using a Draw Hoe

Using a draw hoe is an efficient way to keep weeds at bay in your vegetable patch (or ornamental border). Engaging your deep stabilizing muscles gives your abdominals a workout as you pull the hoe towards you.

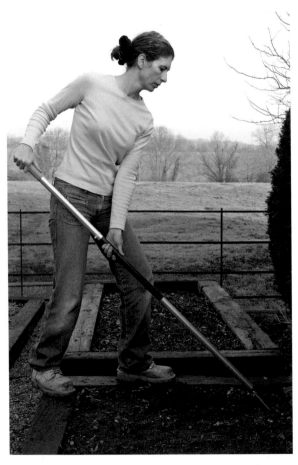

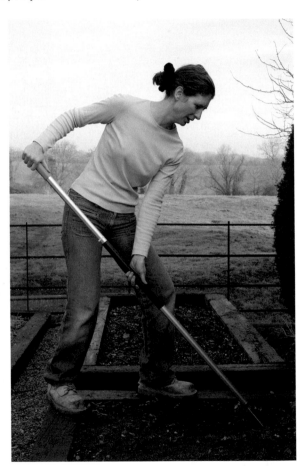

1 Using a long-handled hoe helps you to maintain an upright posture. Begin in a lunge position so that your base is stable. Place your left hand (or, if you are left-handed, your right hand) halfway down the shaft.

2 Then, set your shoulder blades down your back and move the hoe gently back and forth over the soil. The wide-legged stance enables you to shift your weight from foot to foot so that you move with the hoe.

Picking Low

Lowering ourselves down to pick fruits and vegetables is one of those gardening actions that can bring about discomfort and strain, particularly if it is carried out in a way that puts the spine in an awkward position and exerts pressure on the knees.

When picking low, try to avoid staying in one position for sustained periods of time. It really helps to adopt different postures, perhaps alternating between the two positions shown below. If your knees tend to become uncomfortable, try using padded kneelers.

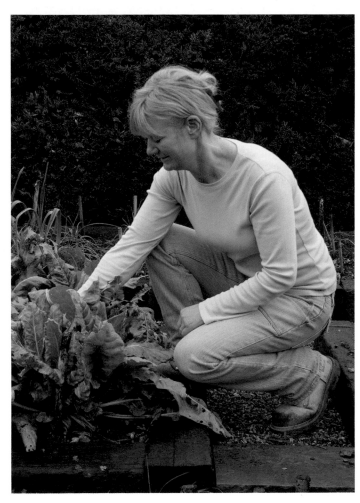

LEFT: When picking crops that are near to the ground, it is best to kneel (unless you have underlying knee problems). However, do not remain in this position for more than fifteen minutes on end.

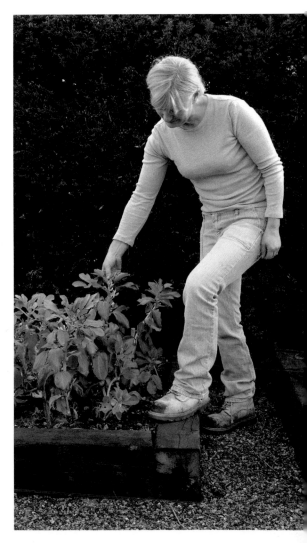

RIGHT: If you find kneeling difficult, remain upright while bending your knees rather than distorting your back. Place one foot forward and try to bend down in a way that lets your spine's natural curves remain largely undistorted. This is, of course, not always possible; sometimes your back may be ever so slightly rounded.

Your Ergonomic Workspace

The exciting powerhouse area of the productive garden, which may include a covered growing area, stock or holding bed, a compost heap, and a potting bench, used to be relegated to bottom of the yard or tucked away out of sight. Yet even in smaller gardens this highly productive area can be arranged for great comfort and designed to look fantastic.

In such a functional area, where plants are continuously moving in and out, an ergonomic design will be a real boon. If you plan the elements of the area to suit your needs, the workspace can feel like a haven. To maximize efficiency and make the most of the time you spend working in it, it helps to site the different elements of your workspace at close quarters.

COVERED GROWING AREAS

It is highly worthwhile to include some form of walk-in, covered growing area in your workspace so that you can remain active and productive in the garden regardless of adverse weather. A greenhouse will help you to produce a great selection of the more tender vegetables such as peppers, tomatoes, and aubergines (eggplants). It also allows you to overwinter tender plants, citrus fruit, brugmansias, and tender perennials such as salvias, widening your repertoire of plants dramatically. Moreover, it is highly convenient for producing streamlined batches of early young seedlings and cuttings to suit your garden's demands. Most gardeners underestimate how much space they will need and then regret that

RIGHT: **This highly functional workspace is always filled with plants moving in and out. It includes compost heaps, mini 'hoarding borders' for growing plants on, glasshouses, potting benches, and areas for standing pots.**

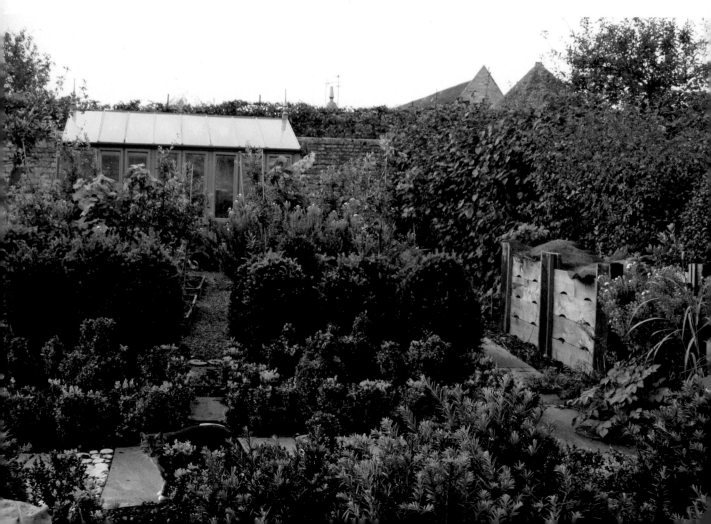

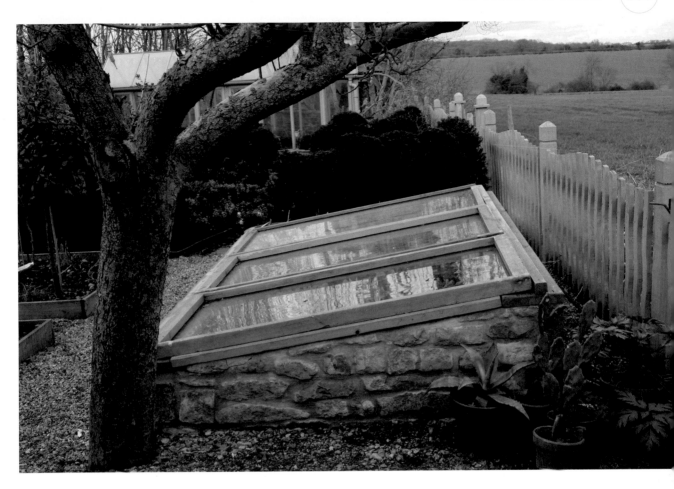

their greenhouse is too small, so if you are investing in one, make sure that it offers ample space.

Polythene tunnels are useful too, and far less expensive—although their big drawback is that they are not nearly as warm as glass structures at night: glass retains the warm air that is radiated from the ground at night, whereas polythene does not, although you can buy treated film which makes it far more efficient. Polythene needs replacing every two or three years—and frankly, it is not exactly beautiful. Rigid polycarbonate is far less brittle than glass but it does not retain the heat. Cold frames, which offer lower-level protection from the elements, are a good alternative to walk-in areas.

Many gardeners get by with no protected space, but the range of crops your garden can produce will increase enormously if you build (or buy) one. When gardeners finally get some covered space, they often wonder how on earth they managed without it!

ABOVE: **This cold frame provides months of fresh, leafy basil and coriander, and is used for rooting cuttings and hardening off plants.**

RIGHT: **Made from reclaimed windows to keep costs down, this greenhouse has been sunk below ground level and stays frost-free (with the help of insulation) throughout the winter.**

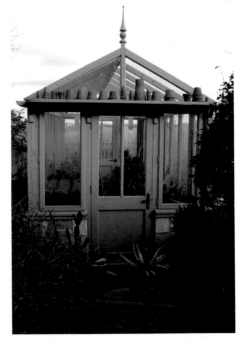

Your Ergonomic Workspace

Postbag editions of BBC Radio 4's 'Gardeners' Question Time' are recorded in this potting shed. A growing sedum roof helps to reduce its impact, and reclaimed scaffold boards clad the sides.

HOARDING OR STOCK BEDS

Hoarding or stock beds enable you to grow young plants in a space where they can be protected from the hurly-burly of life in a grown-up border until they are big and strong enough to thrive in their permanent positions. Young rooted cuttings, plants that you are training up into special shapes, and single specimens that you are using as 'mother' stock from which to propagate can all be arranged in conveniently sized stock beds. If they are raised slightly above ground level for added protection, and small enough to allow you to reach the occupants without treading down the soil, this keeps the soil in good condition even if it regularly disturbed. It is worth filling the beds with the very best soil and compost to give the young plants a strong start. Site these beds in a sheltered part of your working garden, preferably in the sun (netting shading can be slung over shade-loving plants), and arrange the beds' layout so that they look good even when empty.

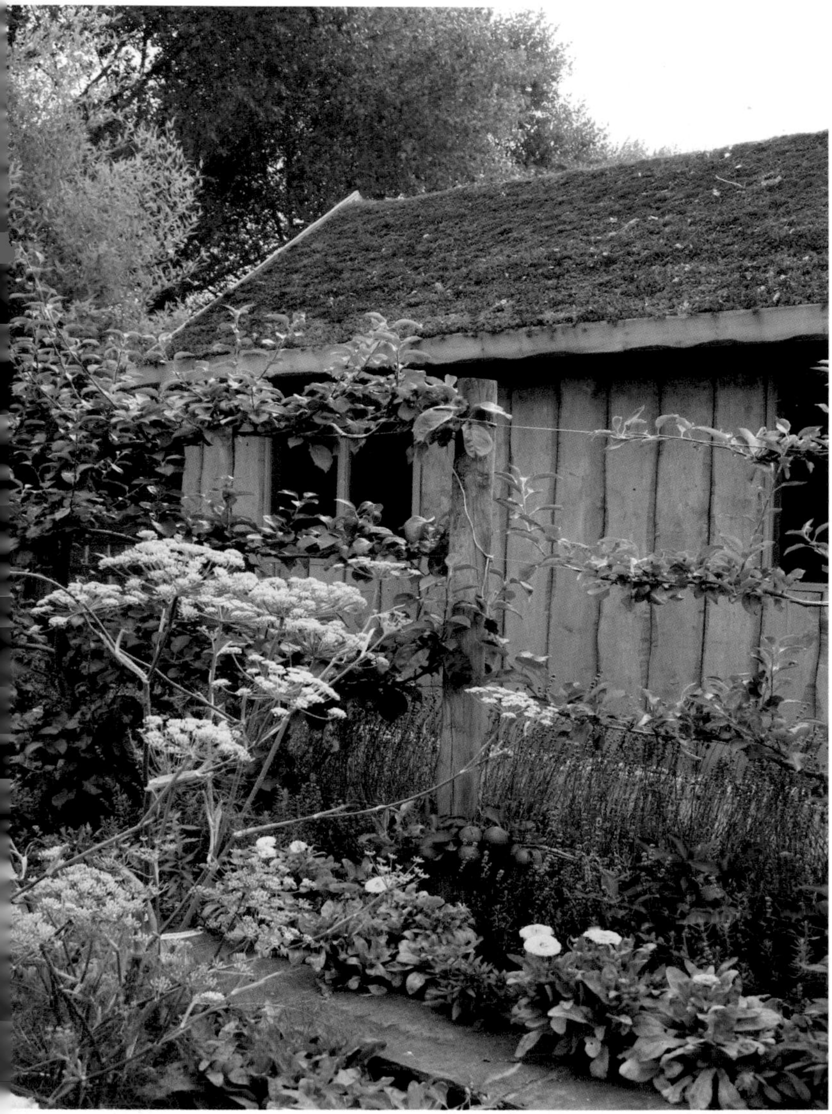

WATER SOURCE

Incorporating a source of water into your workspace is very useful, as it allows you to give your plants a drink (or soak), wash out pots, and dampen the compost heaps. If possible, use a rain barrel that is filled with the rain that collects in your greenhouse and potting shed gutters.

GARDEN SHED

Garden sheds are useful for storing tools, seeds and supplies, and will provide a sheltered space in which to work when the weather is rainy or cold. If it can enhance the overall look of your working garden in addition to being efficiently laid out, then this building may well be your pride and joy.

POTTING BENCH

While some gardeners regard 'potting up' as a chore, others relish it: if your bench is the right height, the sun is on your back, and your compost, pots, and plants are near at hand as you look out over a great garden view, working at a potting bench can be pleasant and relaxing. From a design perspective, an aesthetically pleasing potting bench brings a workmanlike, orderly air to the surrounding area.

When you are producing quite a few of your own plants—vegetables, tender perennials, annuals, shrubs—you soon have to spend significant periods of time pricking out the seedlings, potting them up, and repotting—in short, continually moving them on and up. It is useful to have stocks for replacements and presents, too. You

can then concentrate on standing upright, engaging your core muscles and, of course, doing an excellent job.

The typical height for a work surface is around 3 ft. (90 cm), but the work surface you design should be placed at a height that is very comfortable for you. An easy guide is if you can stand comfortably at your kitchen work surface and that height works for you, then replicate that height. The standard worktop width of around 2 ft. (60 cm) can easily be extended to 2 ft. 3 in. (70 cm) if you have a clear space at the base in which to slot your feet, improving your reach.

If you feel uncomfortable standing for prolonged periods, have limited mobility, or are in a wheelchair, you might consider designing a potting bench that is lower to the ground. A simple tool holder formed from a piece of wood with lugs to hold a hand trowel, fork, and perhaps a walking stick would be useful, as would a tap. It may even be worthwhile to put a roof or an awning over part of the bench, allowing you to remain dry or cool during less favourable weather conditions.

RIGHT: Your work surface should come up to the same height as your waist so that you can stand comfortably to pot; if it is any higher, you may be inclined to lean forward. As you are potting, your back should stay in neutral and if you are standing your knees may bend slightly. Alternatively, you can use a perching seat—just make sure it is low enough that you do not need to lean over to pot.

BELOW: Incorporated into the potting bench is a Belfast sink with taps for washing pots, and plenty of storage space for all of them. A 4-in. (10-cm) timber edge stops compost from disappearing over the sides.

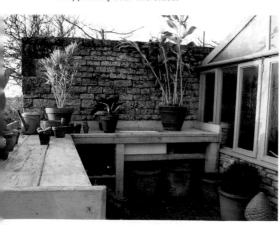

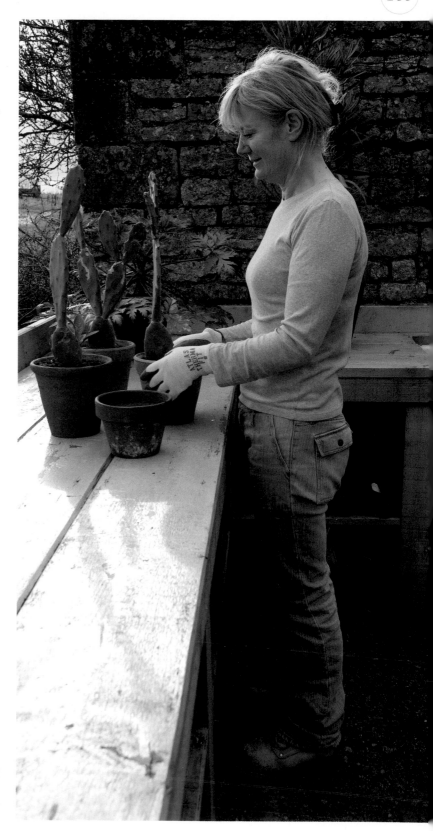

Your Ergonomic Workspace

Lifting Pots Safely

Great plants in pots can lend an opulent, luscious feel to a space. Perhaps this is because the foliage of potted plants tends to be at close proximity to us—almost at eye level, so that it brushes up against our faces. In design terms, the ability to position your potted plants wherever you want offers a fantastic opportunity to manipulate the overall feel of your garden. Adding a few potted 'seasonal specials', such as sensational lilies in pots, is well worth the effort.

When lifting heavy objects like potted plants, your spine can easily become strained. To guard against injury, concentrate on keeping your back in its neutral position as much as possible and focus on taking away some of the strain that would be inflicted on your back by using your legs and abdominal muscles. If your plant has just been watered, the pot will be much heavier than when dry—it makes sense to wait a few days until the water has evaporated before lifting.

1 Squat with your feet apart. Grasp the pot with two hands—never use just one, as this would place a dangerous rotational force on your spine. Bend your knees so that they are pointing outside the pot's edges.

2 As you lift, one foot must remain on the floor to provide a stable base, while the heel of the other foot can come off the floor as you rise to a standing position. The lifting movement should not be too sudden; be sure not to jerk your back or neck.

3 When you stand up, the pot should be grasped firmly with two hands, your shoulder blades should set into your back, and your elbows should be pressed into your sides to maintain your strong grip. While your knees can be slightly bent, your back should remain as straight as possible—do not overarch it. Avoid looking down at the object. Draw strength from your pelvic floor and lower stomach muscles, which should be lifted up and in. Press the heaviest part into your navel.

4 When placing the pot on the table (or any other surface), move your feet into a lunge position with one foot closer to the table so that you avoid having to lean forward.

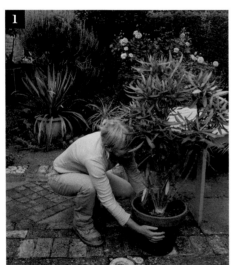

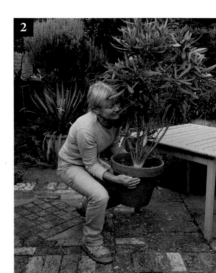

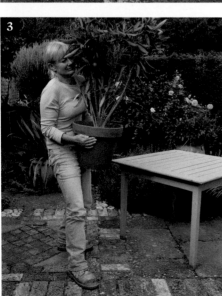

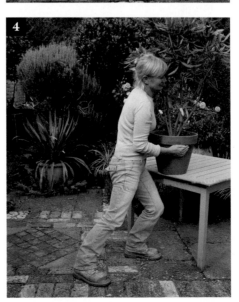

Lifting Alternatives

Before lifting a pot, we must think ahead: is it safe to lift, or is it too heavy? Is the pot slippery? Should a trolley be used? Generally speaking, most pots that are too heavy to lift can be slid onto a little trolley with wheels; if you find that you have to lift many pots, this could be a clever solution. Alternatively, sack barrows can be highly useful. It is sometimes possible to drag the pot on a mat that is quite long, but this is only advisable if the mat is long enough to allow you to keep your spine upright as you drag it across the garden.

However, if these contraptions are somehow not feasible and you find it uncomfortable to bend over to lift up the pot, you can use a nearby sturdy object to support your weight by leaning against it with one hand and using the other hand to lift the pot (but keep in mind that this only works when the pot is light enough to be lifted in one hand). With this method, begin in a lunge stance. If you are lifting with your right hand, place your left leg slightly forward and bent, with the left hand supported on an object or on the thigh. This extra support provided by the object reduces the amount of stress that is placed on your spine. You must be careful not to twist your spine during this process. Again, pull the object close in towards you and use your legs as you lift.

WHO SHOULD AVOID LIFTING HEAVY OBJECTS?

• If you have a back problem, you are probably well aware that you should not put undue strain on your back—so avoid lifting heavy objects like large pots.

• If you have a hip or knee problem you should also exercise extreme caution, as you may not be able to bend your hips and knees enough to avoid placing too much stress on your spine.

• If you suffer from the common condition of a having a rather large stomach, your tummy may prevent you from being able to hold the pot close to your body as you transport it; in this case, call in a helper or simply avoid lifting.

• Finally, if you have a heart condition, a hernia, have had recent stomach surgery, or are pregnant then you should not be lifting heavy objects at all.

Knowing how to lift is important, but it is equally important to know what *not* to do when you lift. Whenever possible, try not to bend at the waist; instead, your legs should be bent as you reach down to grasp the pot. In the first two photos, the back is placed under stress by keeping the knees straight and bending at the waist. As the pot is lifted the back twists. To avoid this, move your feet.

BELOW: These three examples illustrate what not to do when you lift heavy objects.

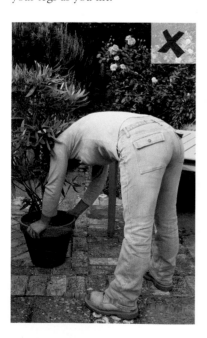
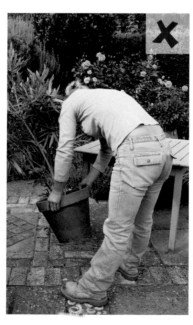
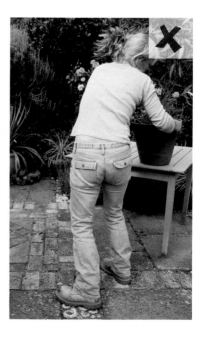

The Compost Heap

A compost heap is a particularly important part of a healthy garden. In addition to the vigorous workout that turning compost gives you, it is a free and nutritious option that saves you from having to lug heavy bags from the nursery or garden centre. It is also environmentally friendly, as it reduces the amount of household waste that goes to landfill sites. Entire books have been devoted to the art and intricacies of producing fine compost, but the truth is that you can put in as much or as little effort as you like.

The more you turn the heap, the more quickly the compost will form. However, if you do not have the time or inclination to turn compost, the material on the heap will probably turn into a good, crumbly compost after about a year if left to its own devices.

TURNING COMPOST

If you want a vigorous aerobic workout, then turning the heap will surely give you one. This is one of the most demanding garden actions.

In essence, turning compost is a full-body workout that requires strength, coordination, balance, and significant strength in your internal 'corset' to support the often strenuous lifting.

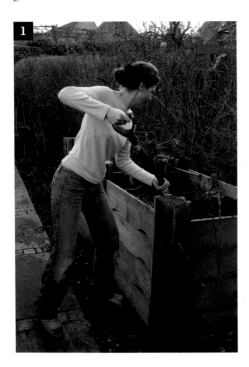

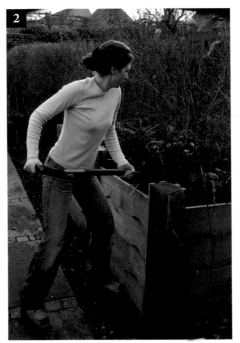

1 Stand with your feet apart so that you can take the weight onto your front leg as you dig into the compost. Your back should remain in neutral, while your shoulder needs to be down, rather than hitched up into your neck. This is hard resistance work, and your whole body will be involved in the movement. Take a moment or two to prepare yourself by lifting your abdominal muscles up and in.

2 As you go to lift the compost up, take more weight onto the back leg and lift your lower abdominal muscles up and in to maintain a neutral spine. Keep your shoulder blade down and in; the exertion of lifting should be felt by the muscles that stabilize your shoulder blades at the back. It helps to make an effort to perform the action from both sides of your body. Alternating sides is very demanding, and will feel strange at first, but it will give you a balanced workout.

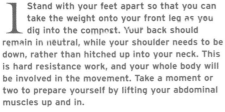

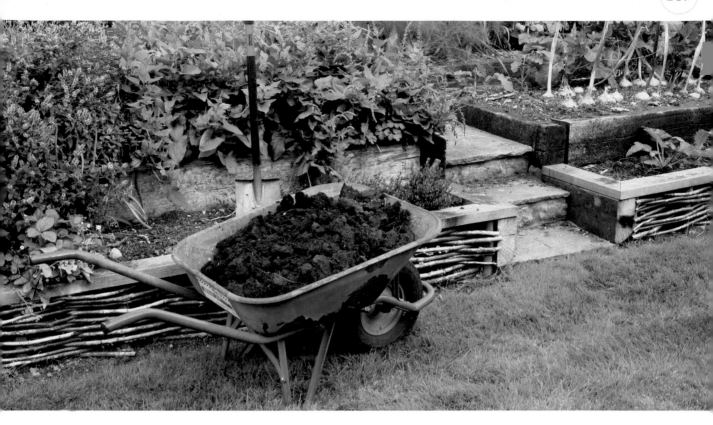

When applied to vegetables during the growing season, compost acts as a mulch to retain moisture as well as improving the soil's humus content.

COMPOSTING TECHNIQUES

Making great compost is rather like baking a great cake: you put lots of different ingredients in, mix it around, then let it bake—and out comes something that bears no resemblance to the raw ingredients. The difference is that with compost-making, you are allowed an infinite number of attempts; if it does not work the first time, you can dig it out, add more greenery, liquid, or activator, and put it back in a heap, and it will improve. Just as cakes provide us with some nutrients, compost feeds your soil. It is especially good for boosting the soil's all-important humus content.

Humus is responsible for creating the soil's texture and structure and gives the topsoil its characteristically dark colour. It is far easier and more rewarding to grow healthy plants on soil with a great structure and high humus content. Conversely, soils that have a low humus content dry out quickly in dry periods to the detriment of the plants. In winter, heavy clay soils with low humus content are easily compacted when worked and tend to become very sticky. Other soils with low humus will have

nutrients rapidly leached through by rain.

We are continually removing plant material like lawn clippings, vegetables, fruit, and weeds from our garden, and composting allows us to put plant matter back. In that sense, it is a sustainable practice. You can also add household waste such as shredded paper to the heap, and recycle your own liquid waste to bump up the volume (which is far better than washing it away with two gallons of clean water every time).

For the beneficial bacteria to work, the ratio of carbon (hard, fibrous material) to nitrogen (soft, green material) should be about 2:1. The 'hard' material is made up of material such as straw or roots, while the 'soft' material is composed of ingredients like green leaves and manures. When you are filling the heap, try to avoid adding a massive chunk of one material in one go. Instead, mix in layers that are no thicker than about 4 in. (10 cm). At times you can be short of green material so use an activator, comfrey leaves, or your own recycled fluid. (If you do not add this material to your heap, it will still form

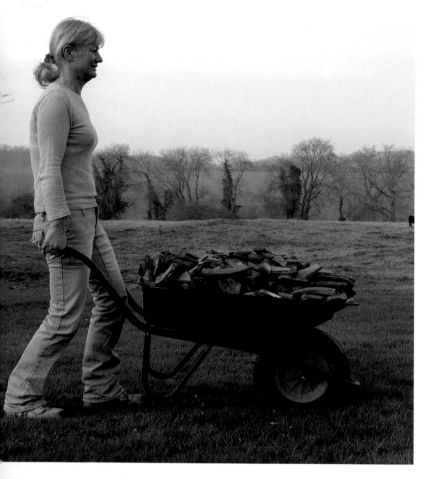

As you push the wheelbarrow, your back should be upright with the spine in neutral, while your arms are slightly bent and your shoulder blades are set down towards the middle of your back. Allow your knees to bend slightly. The muscles in your lower abdominals and arms, rather than your lower back, should take the wheelbarrow's weight as you push it.

greenhouse or polythene tunnel during winter or early spring in order to keep temperatures up. You can sow early tomatoes on top of them and the waste heat will keep off a few degrees of frost. Rats can become attracted to the warm heap and food sources, so they should be lined with protective netting. Add fresh waste every week to ensure that the necessary heat is continuously generated. Rotating bins are also convenient in this situation.

THE FINISHED PRODUCT

When the compost turns a good brown colour, and is sweet-smelling and crumbly, then it is ready to be used. Even if you find the odd bit of cardboard, twig or identifiable object (that lost trowel, for instance!), don't worry—the compost will still be useable.

If you see a white coating that covers much of the material, this indicates that the heap is too dry and is lacking in soft, green material. If you are adding the compost to an area where bulky bits are not acceptable (such as seed beds), sieve the material first and then pop the bulky pieces back onto your heap.

Moving newly made compost gives you a fabulous workout and is especially satisfying on a cold wintry day. During the dormant months it can be difficult to find satisfying aerobic and resistance work, so seize the opportunity and add a barrowload of compost to every square yard (or square metre) of soil that you can. You will see a beneficial change to the soil structure, to the plants and to your body: they will be plumper, while you will be trimmer!

Pushing A Wheelbarrow

Pushing a wheelbarrow—especially one with a heavy load of material inside—is difficult work; it is rather similar to walking on a treadmill at the gym while carrying weights at the same time. The action engages the muscles in your legs, abdominals, arms, and lower back.

It is important to move *with* the wheelbarrow, maintaining control; do not allow it to run away with you so that you have to lean too far forwards to catch up. If you can, avoid leaning over the handles too much. Their height and size should be such that you do not have to stoop over them.

useful compost but will simply take longer). If the material is dry, give each layer a good soak. When the compost bin is full, cover it with some old carpet or similar material to keep it warm. Sometimes your bins never appear to be full (they just shrink when your back is turned), in which case you should just decide when to stop, cover, and then fill another one.

Some materials are best left off the compost heap. They include (but are not limited to) coal, coke ash, cat litter, dog faeces, disposable nappies (diapers), and glossy magazines. Plants with persistent diseases like white rot or club root, perennial weeds, weed seeds, and thick layers of any one material such as grass mowings should also be left off the heap. Large sections of hard wood prunings should be chopped down, burned, or shredded before they are added.

Compost heaps generate a lot of heat, and it can be worth building one in your

Easy and Rewarding Vegetables

If you are really short on time but love the idea of growing your own vegetables, then perennial vegetables should be at the top of your list as they are significantly easier to grow and care for than vegetables that you need to sow, harvest, and remove at least once a year.

In their maintenance demands, the following vegetables are similar to boring, low-maintenance plants like berberis bushes while being significantly more rewarding. Asparagus, globe artichokes, Jerusalem artichokes, seakale, rhubarb, and perennial forms of broccoli and onions are among the easiest vegetables to grow, and they are also the most rewarding; they demand very little maintenance but are reliably nutritious and great-tasting, provided they go into clean soil and are mulched to prevent weeds from germinating. If you are short on time and/ or space, concentrate on those you like best.

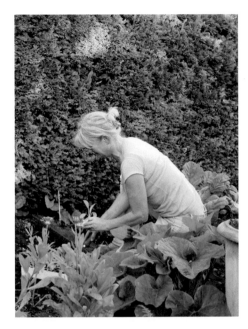

LEFT: Here I am planting vegetable plants that I have grown in modular reuseable polystyrene seed trays. This allows seeds to be sown in a protected environment, away from cats, badgers, and heavy downpours.

BELOW: The amazing organic garden of chef Raymond Blanc at Le Manoir aux Quat'Saisons in Oxfordshire, England, includes vegetables from all corners of the world, including turmeric which is visible in the foreground on the right.

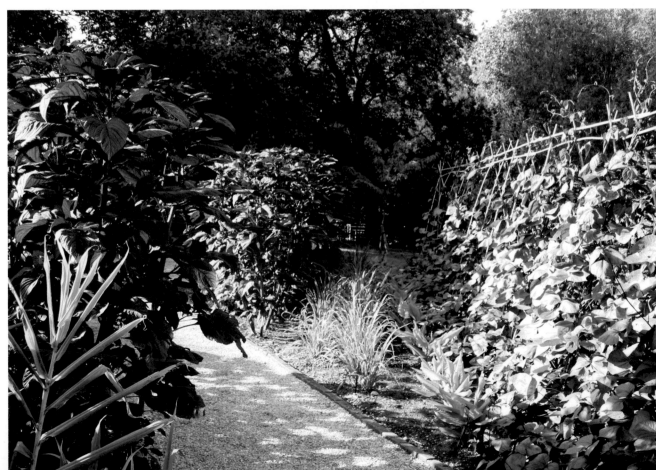

Easy and Rewarding Vegetables

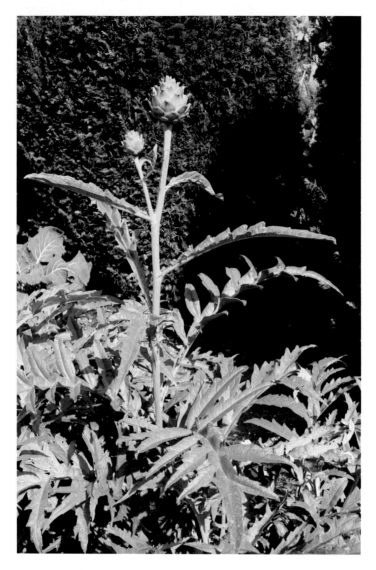

Globe artichokes are attractive, tasty, and easy to grow. With some varieties, the head can be picked when it is as large as a golf ball, and then cooked and eaten whole.

Globe Artichokes

Globe artichokes (*Cynara scolymus*) are fabulous-looking and often considered a delicacy despite being exceptionally easy and prolific. The distinctive, cut, silver-grey leaves that are produced in handsome bold clumps will be largely unscathed in many milder areas in Britain and the United States, and are an eye-catcher throughout most of the year. They definitely deserve a prime position in the ornamental border in addition to the vegetable patch. It is a good idea (and very easy) to take offsets in early spring from a plant known to produce good, succulent heads, as they often do not come true from seed. Some can be less fleshy and harder to eat than others. Although some growers believe that the plants need to be divided every few years to prevent them from becoming congested, others leave them undisturbed for years and still get great results.

Asparagus

It is an old wives' tale that the aristocratic asparagus (*Asparagus officinalis*) demands hard work. Admittedly it is slow to establish—often taking two or three years from planting until you can start cutting the delicious young shoots—but it is well worth the wait. The plants have masses of ferny foliage and turn an attractive butter yellow at the end of the summer. After this, just cut the foliage down. Before planting, make sure that your beds are free of perennial weeds. Give the beds a good, deep mulch each winter.

Perennial Broccoli

In England, the most widely available variety of perennial broccoli (*Brassica oleracea*) is 'Nine Star'. It is useful in that it fills that lean gap in early spring, producing one stout head for picking followed by many smaller, pale green heads. The young leaves can be picked and cooked, too. The plants are tall, and may need staking in windy areas. They are extremely easy to grow from seed, and with luck, they should give you two or three years of produce.

Jerusalem Artichokes

Jerusalem artichokes (*Helianthus tuberosus*) are rarely seen for sale. They are fast-growing, and they do have rampant tendencies. They often reach 6 ft. (2 m) high and are useful for forming a windbreak for your more subdued vegetable plants. The knobbly tubers are quite time-consuming to wash and clean, but it is possible to track down smoother varieties. You can overwinter these plants in the ground in many places. They taste good when roasted around a joint of meat.

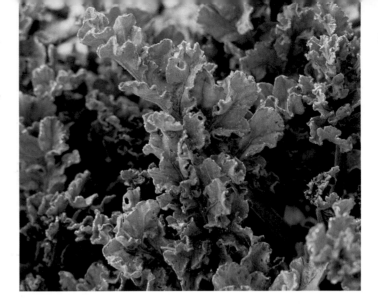

Seakale

Seakale (*Crambe maritima*) is another attractive plant that has large, silvery, slightly crumpled-looking leaves. In midwinter, the plants need to be covered with a buckets or traditional terracotta forcing jars. The young blanched shoots that you pick have an extremely delicate (or bland) flavour. The plants' appearance is generally rated far higher than their taste, but some people are very enthusiastic about this vegetable. As a seaside plant, seakale tolerates wind and performs best on free-draining soils.

Rhubarb

Technically a herb and traditionally eaten as a fruit, rhubarb (*Rheum* species) is nonetheless invariably grown in the vegetable garden. It is extraordinarily easy and its bold, eye-catching leaves and vigorous growth keep most weeds at bay. Rhubarb is enjoying a huge revival now, as its stalks can be made into fabulous sorbets and juices. If you cover the clumps as for seakale, it will give you tender young shoots a few weeks earlier than usual. Drinking rhubarb lemonade is a tasty way to stay hydrated, in the garden or otherwise.

Perennial Onions

The ever-ready onion or scallion (*Allium cepa* 'Perutile') is a perennial alternative to the more traditional onion. It is evergreen and produces delicate clumps about 6–8 in. (15–20 cm) both high and wide. The smaller perennial onions (which you can use as scallions or spring onions) are produced throughout the year. Alternatively, the tree onion (*Allium cepa* Proliferum Group), with clumps of aerial bulbs produced on stalks is a gem: you can eat every part of it.

SELF-SEEDING VEGETABLES

If you do not have the time to sow plants on a regular basis, you should consider choosing some that seed themselves around.

Corn Salad

Corn salad (*Valerianella locusta*; also known as lamb's lettuce) is invaluable in winter salads, tolerates sun or partial shade, and can be cropped twelve months of the year in most areas. Cut the leaves as soon as they are useable; they should re-sprout at least once, and often more. The flowers are edible too, but it is best to leave some to set seed. To stop the self-seeders from appearing too random, consider devoting a whole bed to this bland but useful leaf and occasionally fill in the gaps with replacement seedlings or seeds to keep it looking presentable.

Land Cress

Land cress (*Barbarea verna*), also referred to as American cress, tastes very similar to watercress and is a useful, extremely hardy, low-growing and shiny-leaved biennial that remains green all winter. It will tolerate shade but likes moist, fertile soil, and although it will quickly run to seed in dry conditions, it will self-seed happily in moist conditions. It will re-sprout after cutting, but is slow to do so.

Seakale is an easy and distinctive-looking perennial vegetable. It is quite tasty when eaten raw in salad, and with a few minutes of cooking it complements many dishes.

RHUBARB LEMONADE

8 cups (1.6 kg) rhubarb

3 cups (600 g) brown sugar

3 cups (600 ml) water

3 tablespoons (45 g) lemon zest

1 ½ cups (300 ml) lemon juice, freshly squeezed

Cook the first four ingredients together, and then put through a sieve. When it has cooled, add the lemon juice. To serve, use one part concentrate to three parts water.

Low-Maintenance Fruits and Nuts

Growing fruit is far less demanding than growing most vegetables, and many fruits are well worth including from an aesthetic viewpoint as well as a nutritional one. Fruits are often highly nutritious, with many being high in Vitamin C, roughage, and antioxidants.

If you have enough space in your garden, walnut, hazelnut, sweet chestnut and almond trees are worth including, as they are beautiful to look at and produce nuts that are healthy, tasty, and make excellent quick snacks. Orchards and soft fruit can also look highly attractive, lending the garden a purposeful and productive feel—and they will flourish quite well even if they are not rigorously pruned, sprayed, and tended.

Go for those whose fruits you really enjoy and those that create an atmosphere that strikes a chord with you and fits in harmoniously with the rest of your garden. There is nothing like a mulberry, mature fig, or fruiting lemon tree to endow a garden with a well-established feel. Establishing fruit trees takes a bit of time, but thereafter top fruit will be produced even if the trees are totally neglected.

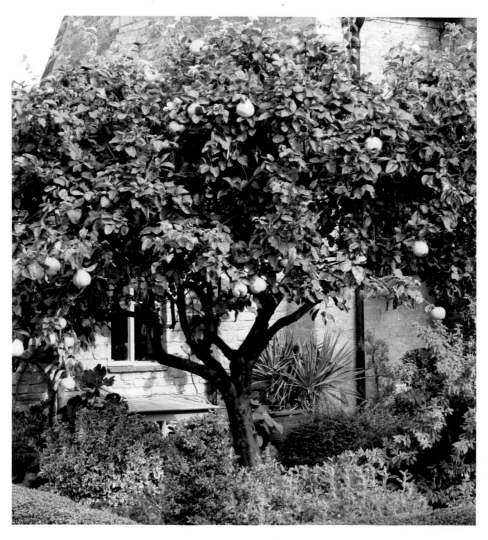

Golden quince fruits look so good on the tree that it can be a shame to pick them. They make a delicious jelly, and add an unusual and fragrant flavour when mixed with apples in crumbles, pies, and tarts.

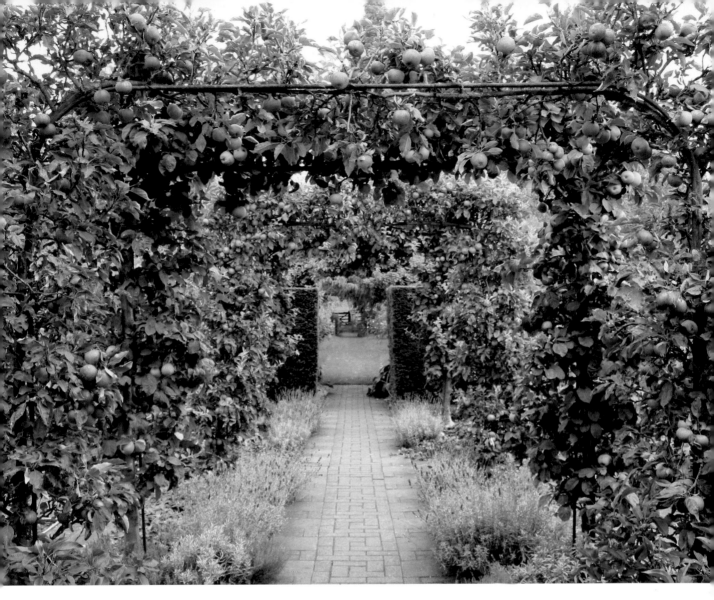

CHOOSING FRUIT TREES

Top fruit is the easiest produce of all to grow successfully. Even if left untended for years at a time, apple and pear trees will often produce satisfying blossom and fruit. They appeal to others, too—birds, bees and many insects thrive among them, adding to the vitality of the garden.

Old gnarled fruit trees look often look decidedly charismatic just as they are, but when you lay out a new orchard you may want to add some design details to lift the space and give it a strong personality. When selecting your trees they are available on different rootstocks with varying degrees of vigour. The less vigorous rootstocks for apples, such as M27 and M9, give rise to small trees that need to be staked throughout their lives. You will never walk under the canopy of these trees, as they are dwarves and their yield is significantly smaller than that of larger trees. On the plus side, they allow you to pick your crop without stretching but you will never create anything like the traditional orchard feel.

The larger rootstocks (MM106 and MM111) will give you trees that establish quickly, give good yields, and will grow to around 12 ft. (4 m). In a small garden, trees trained as espaliers, as step overs, or into goblets are great ways to maximize your use of space and their ornamental nature. Orchards, too, are deservedly popular as they look superb. They help to shelter a garden and create charming, productive, low-maintenance, and useable spaces.

Fruit trees impart a feeling of structure to the garden when grown over archways.

Low-Maintenance Fruits and Nuts

Apples

If you have the space, choose a range of apple (*Malus domestica*) varieties that you cannot buy over the counter. You may want to choose one that has been bred in your local area, or an old-fashioned variety. These may be far tastier than those that you can buy, and although they may have the odd blemish you can still use them for cooking or eating right away—but only the best and most suitable varieties should be stored for

long periods, as not all apples store well. If you are restricted for space, use them in the ornamental garden in place of a specimen tree. They offer a long season of interest, and can be pruned into interesting shapes.

Pears

Strangely, pears (*Pyrus* species) have never been as popular as apples to eat, but their distinctive flavour is a treat and the variability between different varieties is so marked that it is worth seeking out a pear-tasting day at an orchard to decide which ones you enjoy the most. Pear trees are larger and more stately than the trees of many other orchard fruits.

Cherries

If you have room for a cherry orchard, then you are very lucky. Cherries (*Prunus* species) are delicious and contain more Vitamin C and potassium than most other fruits, and they also contain anthocyanins which are believed to be powerful antioxidants. Cherry blossoms are a welcome sight in spring, the striped mahogany trunks are fine, and mature trees make great homes for treehouses as they are not too huge and often have wide spreading branches that accommodate a platform with ease. (To sit up in a canopy surrounded by cherries is fairly tantalizing, too.) If you add a few wild cherries such as *Prunus padus* or *Prunus avium* into a small shelterbelt or copse, you will find that many of the cherries they produce are edible—sweet, but smaller than the fruit of cultivated types. A big bonus is shelterbelt cherries will serve as a 'honey pot' for birds, so they tend to leave other fruit alone.

Quinces

Quince trees (*Cydonia oblonga*) are worthy of being grown on ornamental grounds alone, even if you would never get around to making quince jelly. The early leaves with their felted grey undersides look spectacular, and the papery white blossoms and the golden fruits that follow are eye-catchers. The trees can appear eccentric, but they tolerate pruning and rough shaping.

A FEAST FOR THE EYES

You can add aesthetic appeal to the edible garden by planting fruit trees in an interesting pattern. Geometric shapes work well and enable you to create strong, well-proportioned spaces. To make the pattern more pronounced, you can plant mounds of plants around the base of fruit or nut trees: *Hebe rakaiensis*, *Buxus sempervirens*, and species of *Symphytum* and *Lavandula* are appealing choices. As the trees become larger, their canopies will typically require thinning to allow enough light to get through, but in hot, sunny climates this may not be necessary. If you are mowing under your orchard, a mowing margin of granite setts or other small unit paving in circles or squares around the base of the trunks will stop you from damaging the planting with a mower—and it will also emphasize the design.

Creating walkways through your edible garden will encourage you to use the space. Simple mown paths through longer grass are the simplest to create, but gravel or flagged paths with a network of light metal arches (perhaps used to support arching apples or pears) embellish and define a space.

Grapes

Quite a few new hybrid varieties of grape (*Vitis* species) such as 'Rembrandt' are far more disease-resistant than the older varieties. They are hardy and productive even in cooler climates when planted beside a warm wall. They are also vigorous and extremely useful for creating shade when used to scramble over a horizontal trellis, but if you lack space, the container-grown standards are easy to keep in check by pruning back hard every winter. A potted pair could be used to adorn a gateway or entrance. As ever, fresh homegrown grapes taste far better than store-bought ones (though they may be smaller), and with global warming helping ripening along, a well-sited vine or two are well worth shoehorning into your garden.

Peaches

Peaches (*Prunus persica*) are tasty, but they have the drawback of being prone to peach leaf curl. If you cannot spare the time to spray and cover them with clear polythene early in the year to keep them dry, you should seek out a disease-resistant variety such as 'Avalon Pride', or a dwarf variety such as 'Bonanza' that can be kept under cover in the late winter to mid spring.

Apricots

Apricots (*Prunus armeniaca*) have had much breeding work done on them, and new productive varieties are proving to be very reliable freestanding fruiters. Apricots and peaches flower early in the year when insect activity is low, so it helps to grow some early-flowering plants such as *Symphytum* 'Hidcote Blue' or species of *Vinca* nearby in order to attract bumble bees.

Mulberries

Mulberries (*Morus* species) contain resveratrol, a compound which is thought to reduce the risk of cancer and cardiovascular diseases, and accordingly mulberries are currently being tipped as a new 'super fruit'. The trees are rather large, reaching up to 40 ft. (14 m) or so, but they look magnificent and the fruits make great mulberry gin. If you are short on space, these trees will tolerate pruning or shaping.

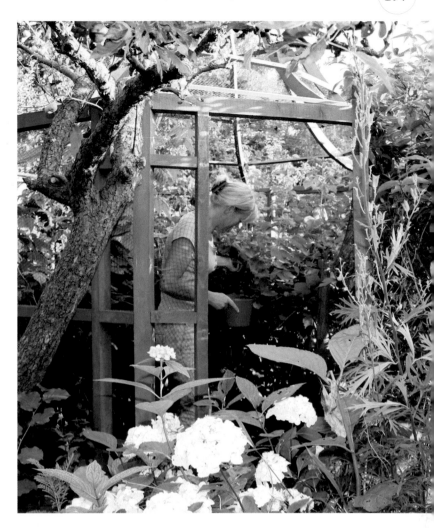

Raspberries can grow well in light shade. Here a homemade fruit cage with curving roof timbers made from plywood ensures that there are raspberries for picking. 'Tulameen' is a high-yielding late summer variety with a superb taste.

SOFT FRUITS

Certain soft fruits demand a little more work than top fruits do, but these are still much easier to cultivate than annual vegetables are. You can always spice up your breakfast cereal with a handful of freshly picked raspberries, currants, or gooseberries or create your own smoothies. It is worth deciding which fruit you crave and rejigging your diet to make sure you can incorporate some freshly juiced berries, or a handful or blackcurrants even if the time to make a sorbet escapes you.

Picking soft fruit is probably the most time-consuming part of the growing process. It is a pleasant task, though, and gives you a great opportunity to unwind at the end of the day, perhaps with a glass of wine or incorporating some bending, stretching, and deep breathing.

Low-Maintenance Fruits and Nuts

Gooseberries

Gooseberries (*Ribes uva-crispa*) are the Cinderella of soft fruit—they tend to be underappreciated, even though they have many advantages. They will fruit even when neglected and will crop even in semi-shade on poor soil. Homegrown gooseberries can be left on the bush until they are really sweet and soft, whereas those available in shops are usually bullet-hard and bitter, and this may be to blame for their relatively unpopularity.

If you have never eaten a ripe, sweet, fresh homegrown gooseberry you will be amazed at its sweet-as-nectar flavour. Whether eaten straight off the bush or in a bowl of cereal, they are high in Vitamin C and contain a lot of healthy roughage. Choose a sweet variety, such as 'Langley Gage', which is white (there are also red and green forms), and grow some early and late forms to lengthen the season.

If you want to use them to adorn your garden in a more upbeat way, you can buy standard gooseberries that are trained on a vertical stem with a neat ball of growth at the top, rather like a deciduous form of a mop head bay. If you plant these in big, attractive pots with their bases removed, allowing them to get their own moisture from the soil below, they certainly earn their keep in any part of the garden.

Alpine Strawberries

Alpine strawberries (*Fragaria vesca*) are easy to grow from seed and do not spread by runners. The fruits are miniscule, but they are extremely tasty and generally ignored by birds. The neat plants form an attractive edge to vegetable beds, and they will produce fruit from early summer to late autumn. They are a real delicacy and work wonderfully as an unusual and tasty garnish for salad, dessert, or cheese.

Raspberries

Raspberries (*Rubus* species) are among the easiest soft fruit to grow. They are packed full of vitamins, and taste sublime. If you do not have time to prepare desserts, just go and graze handfuls from the bushes

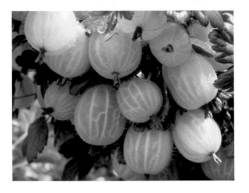

Though they are not as sweet as the pinkish or purplish gooseberries, green gooseberries (which turn golden when ripe) can be sweetened and added to desserts.

with your after-dinner cup of coffee. If you adore salads, a delicious vinaigrette can be made by adding fresh raspberries to the oil and vinegar and then blending it. Recent research has shown that they are high in Vitamin C and antioxidants.

The pruning of the autumn raspberry varieties could not be more straightforward: simply cut all the canes to the ground in late winter. To prevent a weed problem from developing, cover the soil with a deep layer of compost during the winter. The bushes prefer moist, cool conditions so this will also help preserve moisture. Ideally, raspberries should be planted in light shade.

Blueberries

Hailed as 'super fruit', blueberries (*Vaccinium* species) are both sweet-tasting and supremely healthy. They are considered to be one of the richest fruits for antioxidants and research has suggested that they slow the ageing process of some cells. They are also thought to improve short-term memory loss and help with balance and coordination.

Blueberries grow on attractive bushes that require moisture (about 1 in. [25 mm] of rain per week in the growing season), acid soil (with a pH between 4 and 6), and a period of winter chilling in order to crop. It is worth growing them in containers or raised beds if your soil is alkaline, but you should water them from the rainwater barrel and keep a saucer of water underneath their pot.

A mature bush can give you up to 20 lb. (9 kg) of fruit, so they are well worth growing even if your conditions are less than ideal. If your soil is marginal, try planting them in the ground and acidifying your soil annually with sulphur chips. (They may need to be reapplied every six months or so.) Sawdust and regular doses of organic matter will also reduce the pH, making an alkaline soil more acid.

Homegrown blueberries taste far superior to the blueberries available in stores. Wait three days after the berries appear ripe before picking them—they will taste far sweeter.

Currants

Although red, white, and blackcurrants (*Ribes* species) are declining in popularity (perhaps because they can be slightly tart to eat raw and homemade desserts that incorporate currants tend to be extravagant on time and the waistline), they are high in Vitamin C, excellent for making into nutritious juices, and extremely easy to grow. The bushes will tolerate light shade, and all benefit from heavy mulching.

Figs

Known as the 'lazy man's fruit', the common fig (*Ficus carica*) is highly prolific and looks wonderful with its large iconic leaves. Figs are quick to establish and give a garden that wonderful feeling of maturity. Fresh figs are expensive to buy, but they are so easy to grow and when you have a glut you will find that they are tasty with a plate of smoked ham, mixed into salads, or even made into ice cream.

They should be grown either against a wall (generally south-facing is recommended, but in warmer temperatures they can survive and produce reasonable crops whatever their orientation) or as free-standing trees. When grown as trees, be sure to train them up on a leg (or short trunk) to prevent them from forming massive thickets. Alternatively, grow them in a container as a standard tree—they look highly ornamental and fruit well in pots. When planting them in the ground, it is vital to restrict the root growth by planting them in a container with holes; otherwise, they put on too much vegetative growth and fruiting may be reduced.

NUTS
Walnuts

Walnuts (*Juglans* species) have been flying off supermarket shelves as research shows that they are beneficial for the heart; when eaten with saturated fats, they apparently help to block their unhealthy effects. Some people swear by them for arthritis, too, claiming that eating six or seven nuts each day make their symptoms disappear. The fabulous thing about growing your own walnuts is that you can eat them wet (within two to three days of picking), when they are far juicier and have a stronger flavour than they do when dried. You can also pickle the soft green ones after picking in midsummer.

Do invest in a grafted, named cultivar. They are more expensive, but a good one will fruit within a year or two of planting, will flower late (so it is not affected by late frosts), and will be self-pollinating. In England, an excellent, compact walnut tree is 'Rita', which grows to about 25 ft. (8 m) high. Larger ones are 'Broadview' and 'Buccaneer'.

If you have problems with squirrels, place a split, shiny plastic sleeve around the tree trunk, about 4.5 ft. (1.5 m) from the ground and about 3 ft. 8 in. (1.2 m) long. This will be too slippery for the squirrels to climb—but the tree's canopy must be about 9 ft. (3 m) from an adjacent wall or tree to stop them from jumping across.

Sweet Chestnuts

It is worth seeking out newer forms of fruiting sweet chestnuts (*Castanea sativa*) as these will fruit with decent-sized nuts even in cooler climates. These trees tend to fruit three or four years after planting, so it will not be long before you are able to roast your own nuts by the fire. Because most fruiting chestnuts require pollination, you should ideally plant two or three trees. If you have rolling acres, you can coppice these trees by cutting them back to just above ground level every ten years or so. This restricts their height and creates a multistemmed tree, giving you sweet chestnut poles that are highly useful for fencing and firewood.

Almonds

Almonds (*Prunus dulcis*) are tasty, and studies have shown that they can help reduce cholesterol. When you buy almond trees, it is worthwhile to go to a specialist and choose good varieties that are resistant to peach leaf curl. The trees are about 2 ft. (6 m) high, look attractive, and produce a good crop of nuts.

Healthy Herbs

Herbs that you grow in the garden have a variety of different uses. They make tasty and healthy additons to meals, and they also can be used for natural healing remedies.

THE BEST CULINARY HERBS

If you really have precious little time to crop vegetables but you love fresh-tasting food, a selection of high-performing herbs in generous quantities is definitely worth a few square yards (or metres) of border space and a few minutes of tending. If you are pressed for time, buying a bag of mixed leaves and then tossing in some finely chopped tablespoons of fresh lovage, chives, and parsley will produce an original, flavourful salad that does not taste as though it has come straight off the supermarket shelf. Add some chopped fresh thyme leaves to a homemade beef burger and it immediately acquires a sensational twist. Slice some green garlic onto a toasted cheese sandwich and the subtle depth it adds lifts it beyond recognition.

Some herbs, such as parsley, mints, summer savoury, basil, coriander, and lemon balm, are highly useful for culinary purposes but are not particularly ornamental. They respond well to being planted in waves, diagonal lines, or blocks following a checkerboard pattern between paving stones.

Because of the annual, biennial, or shorter-lived nature of many of these herbs, you can afford to be adventurous with your designs. Creating patterns out of blocks of herbs that are contained within low hedging, bricks, woven mini hurdles, or sleepers brings structure and definition to the garden as well as year-round productive areas. If herbs are planted among your vegetables, the flowers and smells will carry the added advantage of confusing pests.

Grow some herbs in large pots to add extra height and interest to the garden. If you garden on wet soils, the well-drained environment of the containers will keep your herbs productive for longer periods. To reduce the need to water them, try removing the bases of the pots and stand them on soil so that they root through to the ground.

Parsley

Parsley (*Petroselinum crispum*) is rich in Vitamins A and C and is a potent antioxidant. It can, however, be awkward to germinate. Watering it in with boiling water after sowing seed along the drill speeds up germination; another option is to germinate it in modules inside first, so that you can safeguard it until it becomes sturdy enough to fend for itself outside. As parsley is biennial, be sure to start sowing the next crop before the last one goes to seed. It is worth covering with a cloche in hard winter weather, to ensure a winterlong supply.

Mint

Mint (species of *Mentha*) has a reputation for being contrary. Some gardeners have difficulty containing mint plants because they are so invasive. (If you find that this is the case, try confining them to a pot or bottomless container sunk into the ground.) Confoundingly, other gardeners claim to be unable to grow mint at all. Mints prefer moist soils, so this may be the key; mint plants should be watered copiously until they are well established. They are of course highly valuable in the kitchen, and an excellent remedy for indigestion. *Mentha spicata* var. *crispa* 'Moroccan' has a superb spearmint flavour that is great for tea.

Summer Savoury

Summer savoury (*Satureja hortensis*) is a useful culinary herb especially suitable for salt-free diets. It is believed to be especially beneficial for pregnant women.

Basil

Basil (*Ocimum basilicum*) is a highly popular cooking herb, superb in pesto and salads. The plant is an easy annual that thrives in warm conditions; it is such a winner that it is worth growing it in the ground in a cold frame or under a mini polythene tunnel during the summer, to guarantee a mass for many months each year even if your summer weather is not particularly warm. Experiment with such fabulous varieties as the highly attractive purple basil (*Ocimum basilicum* var. *purpurascens*) and bush basil (*Ocimum minimum*) which has leaves half the size of ordinary basil, and bushier growth.

Coriander

Coriander (*Coriandrum sativum*) has the reputation of bolting—going straight up to seed without giving you the sought-after, wonderfully tasty leaves. To prevent this, avoid moving the plants, or keeping them too dry; they should be well-watered, especially in very hot conditions. It is also worth seeking out varieties that have been specially bred for longer leaf production: 'Confetti', 'Leisure', 'Slow Bolt', and 'Santo' are all high-performing choices.

Lemon Balm

Lemon balm (*Melissa officinalis*) is prone to looking rather weedy, like a nettle, after its first flush of growth, and it tends to seed around. Yet it is now being looked at in a more favourable light, perhaps due in part to its supposed health benefits. In a study carried out in 2003 at England's Northumbria University, lemon balm was found to increase the activity of acetylcholine, an important chemical messenger linked to memory, that is reduced in people with Alzheimer's disease. It appears to improve the ability to learn, store, and retrieve information, and in this study the herb improved the mood of the volunteers by inducing calmness. In these trials dried leaf was used, but an infusion of leaves in boiling water could be substituted.

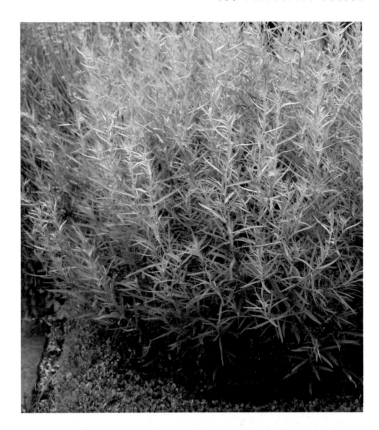

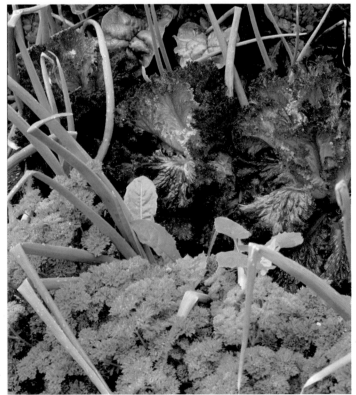

ABOVE RIGHT: Tarragon prefers poor soil and is a very easy perennial herb to grow. This is Russian tarragon, which has a milder flavour than French tarragon, and is tasty in salads.

RIGHT: Parsley growing in a compact row alongside other herbs and bright lettuces makes for a colourful display.

Healthy Herbs

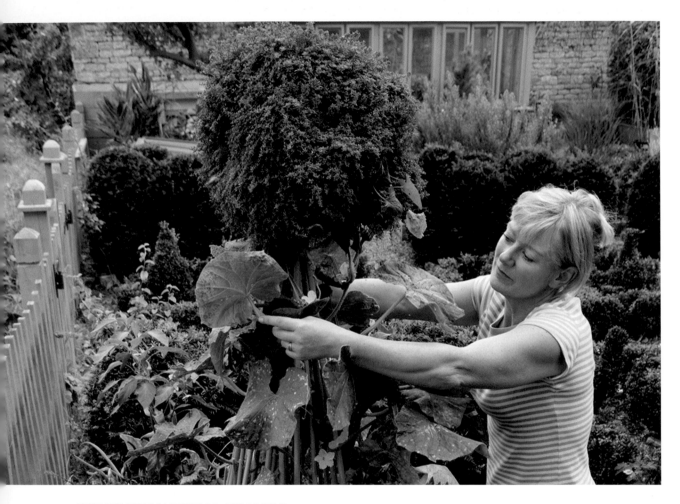

HERBS FOR NATURAL HEALING

Herbs have been used for millennia to improve all sorts of conditions, and now modern research has been backing up many of the traditional claims to healing. Aromatherapy has played a role in communities around the world since ancient times (evidence suggests that the Egyptians distilled fragrant essential oils for cosmetic and medicinal use as long ago as 4500 BC), but it was not until 1937 that the French scientist René Maurice Gattefossé researched the healing potential of essential oils and coined the term 'aromatherapy' after conducting research into the healing potential of essential oils.

In the 1950s, an Austrian surgical assistant named Marguerite Maury began to blend the oils to suit the needs of individual patients, spurring more widespread interest in aromatherapeutic formulations as a viable alternative way of treating a range of different conditions, from depression and anxiety to migraine headaches.

The following herbs are really worth spending a few more minutes on tending, so you can make your own organic solutions whenever you feel tensed up (or even increasingly forgetful). In addition to their natural healing benefits, these herbs are also desirable for their culinary and aesthetic qualities.

Peppermint

Peppermint (*Mentha ×piperita*) may be used be in cold compresses for joints as it has an

This raised container produces a good range and high volume of herbs and vegetables. Parsley and basil are grown among the tomatoes, lettuces, cucumbers, purple French beans, chilli peppers, and onions. A ball of thyme sits on top of the painted canes.

analgesic quality. (It is therefore good to have peppermint on hand in case you sprain yourself in the garden.) If you infuse the leaves for five minutes and drink this after a meal, it is believed to help relieve indigestion.

Sage

Sage (*Salvia lavandulifolia*) has a longstanding reputation for enhancing memory and recent research has shown that the scent of Spanish sage (in the form of essential oil) significantly improved word recall. It is also supposed to be good for menopausal problems such as hot flashes, but should be used with caution as it may be toxic when taken in excess over long periods. Many herbalists believe *Salvia officinalis* 'Purpurascens' to be more potent than the species.

It is excellent for cooking, too—and if you boil sage in water (perhaps adding some peppermint and rosemary), it makes a good mouthwash. The broadleaved form (*Salvia officinalis*) has the bonus of lending an all-year-round sense of structure to the garden.

Thyme

The larger, bushier forms of thyme (*Thymus* species) are valued as attractive edging, and thyme is also indispensable for culinary and therapeutic use. (To quickly remove leaves from stalks, cut the stalks and put them in a bag in the freezer for few hours; you will then be able to easily shake off the leaves.) Clinical trials have supported the use of thyme to help treat productive coughs, and an infusion of thyme sweetened with honey is a traditional remedy for whooping cough, sore throat, and catarrh.

Angelica

Angelica (*Angelica archangelica*) is a fabulously ebullient, 6.5-ft. (2-m) high biennial. Just let it seed and produce new plants from its umbels of beautiful flowers. A hot, aqueous infusion of aniseed, cinnamon, fennel, ginger, garlic, and angelica was traditionally taken to counteract catarrhal congestion.

Borage (Starflower)

In wilder areas, the forget-me-not blue flowers of borage (*Borago officinalis* or *Echium amoenum*), are a dream. Be careful, though, as they prone to taking over! Add leaves to summer drinks to impart cucumber flavour. Borage's leaves, flowers, and seeds are believed by some herbalists to help counteract feelings of melancholy.

Myrtle

Myrtle (*Myrtus communis*) is a beautiful, evergreen bush that thrives in sheltered spots. It grows to 13 ft. (4 m) but can also be kept much smaller, and it withstands clipping very well.

The myrtle is a symbol of peace, love, and happiness and it is often given as a wedding present. It emits a fabulous fragrance from its white flowers and its leaves are excellent additions to pork and lamb dishes. Myrtle oil is a main ingredient in Gelomyrtol, a product prescribed to treat bronchitis and sinusitis.

GROWING, HARVESTING, AND STORING HERBS

The finest herbs are those that you can pick when there is not much else around. An ideal place to keep herbs is on a windowsill inside the house. If your sills are deep enough, it is worth getting custom-made, shallow, galvanized metal trays to stand your mix of pots in to help contain any stray water, and use every square inch or centimetre available. Copper, lead, zinc, and iron are available in sheet form and they are simple to form into a smart-looking tray, ideal for adorning kitchens and conservatories, providing you with rich pickings throughout the year. Greenhouses and cold frames are obvious places to grow herbs, and cloches are ideal for those without these structures.

When harvesting your herbs, collect small quantities at a time and handle them with care. If you can smell their fragrance while you are picking them, this means that you are losing some of their valuable, volatile oils. Only collect one herb at a time, and pick only from healthy plants that are in good condition. If you are storing herbs, cut them on a dry, sunny morning after any rain or dew has evaporated.

When you have a glut of herbs, it is worth storing the best ones. There are different ways to preserve herbs: drying, freezing, making herb juices and pastes, making herb oils or vinegars, and preserving in sugar. Drying is most common, but do not ignore other methods. Basil leaves are divine packed in oil—the leaves can then be used in sauces, and the oil is fantastic for dressings. Herb juices that involve liquidizing the herbs and, if required, freezing the juice, can be useful. However, keep in mind that a great many leaves will yield only very small quantities of juice.

Healthy Herbs

Coneflower (Echinacea)

Coneflower (*Echinacea purpurea*) is a showy, long-flowering plant that is valued as much for its eye-catching flowers as for its herbal properties. Clinical trials have supported its use for a range of conditions; in particular, echinacea is believed to be very effective in boosting the immune system. For best results, try to keep slugs well away.

Golden Oregano

A compact plant with striking yellow foliage, golden oregano (*Origanum vulgare* 'Aureum') has been found by the American National Cancer Institute to have modest anticarcinogenic properties along with the mints, rosemary, thyme, sage, and basil.

Feverfew

An attractive perennial with single white flowers, feverfew (*Tanacetum parthenium*) has the pleasant habit of seeding itself around; it will slot itself into even the tiniest crevice. A small amount may be added to food to cut down on grease. It also may be effective as a treatment for migraine; in one series of trials, 72% of all the participants found that their condition improved and the associated nausea and vomiting decreased or disappeared. The part used medicinally is the leaf collected when the plant is in flower. Many users take fresh leaves, usually about three per day, often in a sandwich. (If you are pregnant, this should be avoided.)

Lavender

The scent of lavender (*Lavandula angustifolia*) is strongly believed to have a relaxing, and even sedative, effect. Keep a few sprigs up your sleeve for deep breaths whenever you are feeling nervous; it really has an amazing calming effect, yet it is also likely to boost your mood. If you mix dried lavender sprigs with olive oil and simmer for few hours, this is believed to help alleviate spots, bites, rashes, and sunburn.

Echinacea purpurea 'Rubinstern' has intense carmine-red petals that are beautifully horizontal.

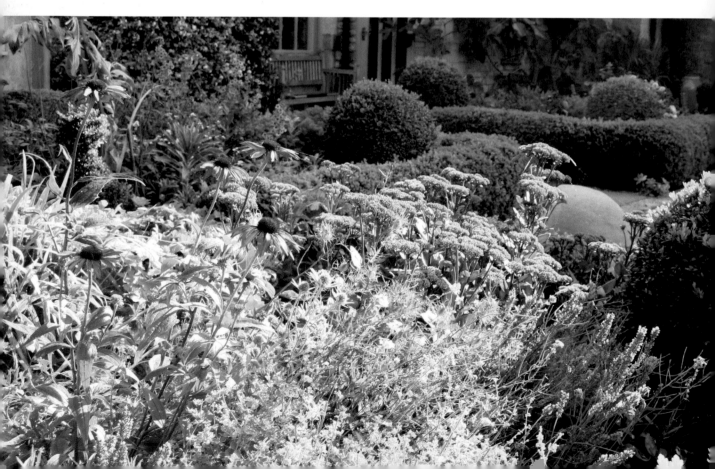

Lavender plants look wonderful when used to form generous sweeps and hummocks. Free drainage and sun are vital; otherwise, it can look miserable. Prune hard after flowering (but no later than late summer) to prolong bushiness.

Rosemary

Rosemary (*Rosmarinus officinalis*) is a quick-growing plant that is well suited to growing as topiary as well as in pots. Its welcome blue flowers are frequently produced in the winter months. It is thought to be the original Christmas tree, used long before the Norway spruce, and it is believed that if rosemary is brought into the house on Christmas Eve you will have good luck for the rest of the year. The flowers of rosemary are tasty; try tossing some in with runner beans to accompany lamb.

One study has suggested that rosemary oil may be a highly beneficial stimulant. Inhalation and oral administration of rosemary oil has been shown to bring about noticeable improvement in the locomotor activity of mice. Rosemary essential oil is recommended for the relief of rheumatism and tired, overworked muscles—an ideal treat after a hard day of work in the garden.

LAVENDER LEMONADE

¼ cup (50 g) fresh lavender blooms

1 cup (200 g) sugar

5 cups (1 litre) water

Juice of 1 freshly squeezed lemon.

Mix the sugar with 2 ½ cups (500 ml) of water. Bring it to a boil, stirring to dissolve the sugar. Then, remove from the heat and add the lavender flowers to the hot syrup.

Leave to steep for several hours, before straining and removing the solids. Add the lemon juice and the remaining water. Serve chilled on ice with a few sprigs of fresh lavender to garnish.

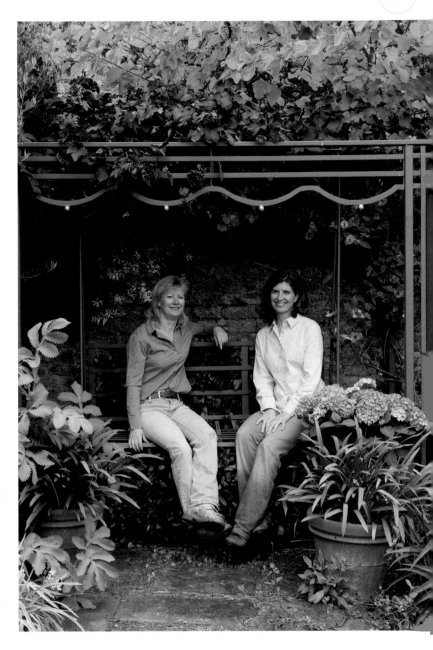

Few gardeners take the time to just sit and relax in the garden, perhaps because we tend to feel there is always room for improvement. Make sure that you get around to making use of your sitting areas—relaxation is a vital part of the fit gardener's regime!

ACKNOWLEDGEMENTS

Firstly thanks are due to Anna Mumford, who commissioned the book, and to Erica Gordon-Mallin, the editor, for all of her sterling work and enthusiasm; to Bridgewater Books, who designed the book; and of course to Colin Leftley for the many step-by-step sequences and other photographs. We are also grateful to Marianne Majerus, Marie O'Hara, and Kevin Guinness for all their early morning rises and great photographs.

We would also like to thank the following who have allowed us to photograph their gardens: Stapleford Park Hotel, Val Jackson, Paul and Ros Evans-Flagg, The Late Prince and Princess Galitzine, Terry and Susan Symons, Raymond Blanc and Le Manoir Aux Quat'Saisons, Sue and Jon Wimpeney, Helen Dillon, Susie and Ian Pasley-Tyler, Mr. and Mrs. Akio Shoji and Aleph Inc., Annie Huntindon, Francesca and Philip Kendall, Sparsholt College, Cleve West, Bas and Jane Clarke, Stephen Cooke and Nia Morris, Professor Peter and Doctor Sarah Furness, Mary and Miles Napier, Mr. Barry Townsley and the Right Honourable Laura Townsley, and Robert and Beverley Murphy. We must also thank in particular Kate King for helping in the garden.

Robbie Philp of the Pilates Studio in Peterborough has been extremely helpful and he has a gift for making Pilates fun and fascinating. Thanks are also due to Enzinga Pele for her fitness and Pilates instruction. Professor Clyde Williams, Professor of Sports Science at Loughborough University, has provided much invaluable information and Polar have provided calorie-counting and heart rate monitor watches. We also owe our thanks to Wilkinson Sword Garden Power Tools and Colin Berridge of Peterborough Garden Machinery for lending us some equipment, and to Barlow Tyrie for lending us some garden chairs.

Finally, I (Bunny) would like to thank my long-suffering family, and Karen Harvey and Zoë Traherne for their help with shots

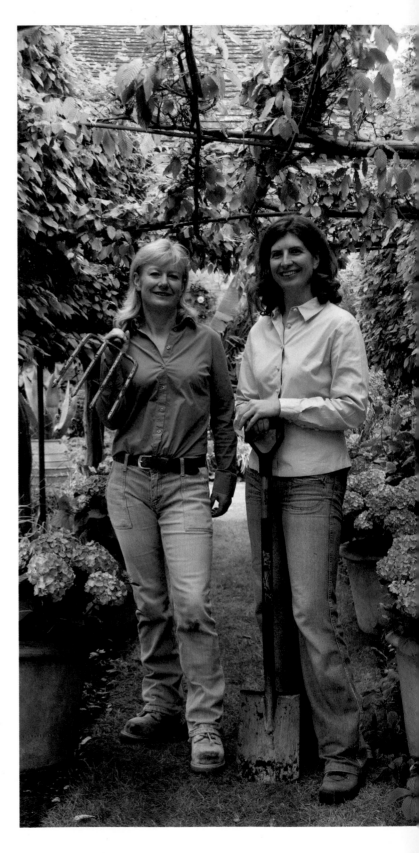

REFERENCES

Bradley, Dinah. *Hyperventilation Rehabilitation: Breathing Patterns Disorders and How to Overcome Them.* LONDON: Kyle Cathie Limited, 1998.

Carr, Janet and Roberta Shepherd. *Neurological Rehabilitation: Optimizing Motor Performance.* OXFORD, UK AND WOBURN, MASSACHUSETTS, USA: Butterworth-Heinemann, 1998.

Carrière, Beate. *The Swiss Ball: Theory, Basic Exercises, and Clinical Applications.* NEW YORK: Springer Publishing Company, 2000.

Franklin, Eric N. *Dynamic Alignment Through Imagery.* LEEDS, UK AND CHAMPAIGN, ILLINOIS, USA: Human Kinetics, 1996.

Kovar K. A., B. Gropper, D. Friess, and H. P. T. Ammon. 1987. *Blood levels of 1,8 cineol and locomotor activity of mice after inhalation and oral administration of rosemary oil.* PLANTA MEDIA 53: 315–318.

Maughan, R. J. (ed.). *Nutrition in Sport.* OXFORD: Blackwell Publishing, 2000.

Mills, Simon and Kerry Bone. *Principles and Practice of Phytotherapy: Modern Herbal Medicine.* LONDON: Churchill Livingstone, 1999.

Oliver, Jean. *Back Care: An Illustrated Guide.* Burlington, MA: Butterworth-Heinemann, 1994.

Pandrangi, S. and L. F. LaBorde. 2004. *Retention of folate, carotenoids, and other quality characteristics is commercially packaged fresh spinach.* THE JOURNAL OF FOOD SCIENCE. 69: 702–707.

Roberts, Matt. *Fitness for Life Manual.* LONDON: Dorling Kindersley, 2002.

Robinson, Lynn, Helge Fisher, Jacqueline Knox, and Gordon Thomson. *The Official Body Control Pilates Manual.* LONDON: Macmillan Publishers Ltd., 2000.

Scholey, Andrew and David Kennedy. 2003. *Modulation of mood and cognitive performance following acute administration of single doses of lemon balm.* NEUROPSYCHOPHARMACOLOGY 28: 1871–1881.

APPENDIX

High-Quality and Ergonomic Gardening Tools

Mecanaids, Inc.
21 Hampden Drive
South Easton, Massachusetts
02375 United States
T (800) 227-0877
F (508) 238-1752

PETA (UK) Ltd.
Mark's Hall
Mark's Hall Lane
Margaret Roding
Dunmow CM6 1QT
United Kingdom
T 01245 231118
F 01245 231811
www.peta-uk.com

Sneeboer
⅝ Cole Gardens
430 Loudon Road
Concord, New Hampshire
03301 United States
T (603) 229-0655
F (603) 229-0657
www.sneeboerusa.com

Wilkinson Sword Garden Power Tools
Fiskars Brands UK Ltd.
Newlands Avenue
Bridgend CF31 2XA
United Kingdom
T 01656 655595
F 01656 659582
www.wilkinsonswordgarden.co.uk

Garden Clothing and Accessories

Aigle (Wellington boots & gardening clothes)
⅝ Dillard's Corporate Headquarters
1600 Cantrall
Little Rock, Arkansas
72201 United States
info@aigleusa.com
www.aigleusa.com

Keane Gardeneur (thin gloves)
P.O. Box 44355
London SW20 0XB
United Kingdom
T 020 8946 8522
www.keanegardeneur.co.uk

Muck Boot Co. (Eden shoes)
74a Wellington Road
Turton, Bolton BL7 0EG
United Kingdom
T 01204 853852

Skillers Workwear
299-A Washington St.
Woburn, Massachusetts
01801 United States
T (781) 933-5400
F (781) 933-5420
www.skillers.com

Snickers Original
Unit N3 Gate 4
Meltham Mills Industrial Estate
Meltham, Holmfirth HD9 4DS
United Kingdom
T 01484 854488
www.snickersdirect.co.uk

Miscellaneous Supplies For Easier Gardening

Agralan Limited (protective meshes for vegetables)
The Old Brickyard
Ashton Keynes
Swindon, Wilts SN6 6QR
United Kingdom
T 01285 860015
www.agralan.co.uk

Enstone Breedon Ltd. (bound gravel)
Breedon on the Hill
Derby DE73 1AP
United Kingdom
T 01332 862354

Lindum Wildflower (ready-grown wildflower with turf, grown on felt)
West Grange, Thorganby,
York, YO19 6DJ
United Kingdom
T 01904 448675
www.turf.co.uk

Rainharvesting Systems (irrigation supplies)
The Greenshop
Cheltenham Road
Bisley, Stroud, Glos GL6 7BX
United Kingdom
T 08452 235430
www.rainharvesting.co.uk

Tenax Corporation (fabric membranes)
4800 East Monument Street
Baltimore, Maryland
21205 United States
T (410) 522-7000
F (410) 522-7015
www.tenaxus.com

Tildenet Ltd. (fabric membranes)
Hartcliffe Way
Bristol BS3 5RJ
United Kingdom
T 01179 669684

Garden Design

Bunny Guinness Landscape Design
www.bunnyguinness.com

North American Sources for Hard-to-Find Gooseberries and Currants (Chapter 6)

Al Eppler Inc.
Box 16513
Seattle, Washington
98116 United States
T (206) 932-2211
Edible Landscaping
361 Spirit Ridge Lane
Afton, Virginia
22920 United States
T (434) 361-9134
F (434) 361-1916
www.ediblelandscaping.com

Gourmet Acres
1439 Sale Barn Road
Greely, Ontario
K4P 1L6 Canada
T (613) 821-1345
F (613) 821-0970

Foam Rollers, Weighted Balls, Mats, and Other Exercise Equipment

Balanced Body Pilates Equipment
8220 Ferguson Avenue
Sacramento, California
95828 United States
T (800) 745-2837

The Physical Company,
2a Desborough Industrial Park,
Desborough Road
High Wycombe, Bucks, HP12 3BG
United Kingdom
T 01494 769222

Heart Rate Monitors and Calorie-Counting Watches

Polar Electro
Polar House,
Heathcote Way, Unit L
Heathcote Industrial Estate
Warwick, Warwickshire CV34 6TE
United Kingdom
T 01926 310330
www.polarelectro.co.uk

Polar USA
1111 Marcus Avenue, Ste. 115
Lake Success, New York
11042 United States
T (516) 364 0600
www.polarusa.com

Resources for Wellbeing

The American Physical Therapy Association (APTA)
1111 North Fairfax Street
Alexandria, Virginia
22314 United States
www.apta.org

Back Care
www.backcare.org.uk

Barnhouse Physiotherapy
Main Road, Tallington
Stamford, Lincolnshire PE9 4RP
United Kingdom
T 01780 740242
www.barnhousephysio.co.uk

Body Control Pilates
35 Little Russell Street
London WC1A 2HH
United Kingdom
www.bodycontrolpilates.com

The Disability Information Trust
Mary Marlborough Centre
Headington, Oxford, OX3 7LD
United Kingdom
T 01865 227592
F 01865 227596

Horticultural Therapy Institute
P.O. Box 461189
Denver, Colorado
80246 United States
T (303) 388-0500
www.htinstitute.org

**Planet Amber
(health and disability resources)**
www.planetamber.com

Robbie Philp (Pilates instruction)
4 Dodson Way
Vitas Business Park
Boongate. Peterborough PE1 5XG
United Kingdom
T 07732 632671

ENERGY TABLE

Using this table, you can work out a more precise number of calories burned per hour for a variety of different activities based on your body weight. For instance, if you weigh 112 pounds (8 stone) and want to calculate the amount of calories used when you lay turf for one hour: multiply 2.3 × 112, giving you a total calorie consumption of 257.6. The metric equivalent can be calculated in the same way. (Adapted from *Nutrition in Sport.*)

Activity	Calories used over 1 hour per kg body weight	Calories used over 1 hour per pound body weight
Driving fast	1.9	0.9
Light office work	1.4	0.6
Lying in bed, quietly, awake	0.9	0.4
Sitting watching television	0.9	0.4
Standing, quietly	1.2	0.5
Carrying heavy loads, e.g. large pots	7.8	3.5
Carrying, loading, or stacking wood	5.0	2.3
Carrying logs	10.9	4.9
Chopping logs with axe, fast-paced	16.9	7.7
Chopping logs with axe, slow-paced	5.0	2.3
Chopping wood, splitting logs	5.9	2.7
Clearing land, hauling branches	5.0	2.3
Collecting grass or leaves	4.0	1.8
Digging, spading, filling garden	5.0	2.3
Gardening with heavy power tool, tilling a garden	5.9	2.7
Laying hardcore, crushed rock	5.0	2.3
Laying turf	5.0	2.3
Mowing lawn, hand mower	5.9	2.7
Mowing lawn, power mower	4.5	2.0
Mowing lawn, riding mower	2.4	1.1
Operating snow blower, walking	4.5	2.0
Planting seedlings or shrubs	4.0	1.8
Planting trees	4.5	2.0
Raking lawn	4.0	1.8
Shovelling snow by hand	5.9	2.7
Shovelling, digging ditches	8.3	3.8
Shovelling, heavy	9.0	4.1
Shovelling, light	5.9	2.7
Shovelling, moderate	6.9	3.1
Spreading soil with shovel	5.0	2.3
Trimming shrubs or trees with power trimmers	3.6	1.6
Trimming shrubs or trees with shears (secateurs)	4.5	2.0
Walking, applying fertilizer or seeding lawn	2.4	1.1
Watering lawn or garden	1.4	0.6
Weeding	4.5	2.0

INDEX

Page numbers in italic type refer to picture captions.